To my friend Jean with very best wishes with admiration Roberta Crawford

The Iron Elephant

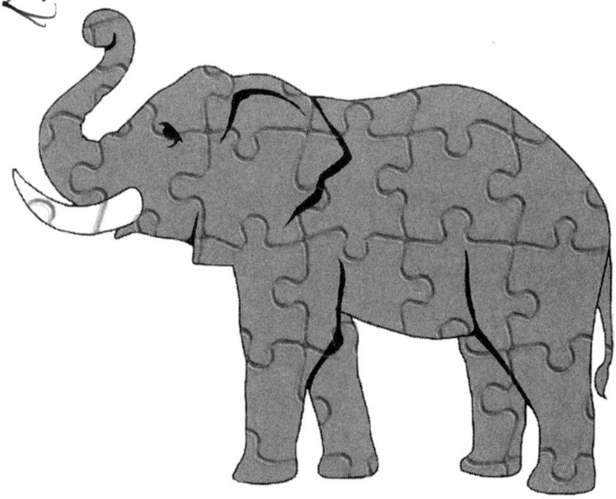

The Iron Elephant

What You Should Know
About The Danger
Of Excess Body Iron

Roberta Crawford

Vida Publishing, Inc.

P.O. Box 296

Glyndon, MD 21071-0296

 For information address Vida Publishing, Inc., PO Box 296, Glyndon, MD 21071-0296.

SECOND EDITION

FIRST PRINTING - May 1992
SECOND PRINTING - March 1993

SECOND EDITION - UPDATED - EXPANDED
FIRST PRINTING - January 2000

Cover by Kathleen Minacapelli
Library of Congress Catalog-in-Publication Number 98-60879

Crawford, Roberta
The Iron Elephant/Roberta Crawford 2nd ed.

ISBN 0-9632547-7-4 (pbk)
1. Health—Popular works. I. Title

Dedicated to the hundreds of physicians around the world and to the directors, members and faithful volunteers of Iron Overload Diseases Association, Inc., whose support and caring have helped the organization thrive, and who made this book possible.

This book is intended to help the reader look at iron with new eyes, to see iron in a new light, and to gain understanding of the proper place of iron in human health. This book should not be substituted for the advice and treatment of a physician but rather should be used as enhancement of the reader's understanding of iron. The author and publisher disclaim responsibility for any adverse effects resulting from the information presented here.

Contents

Preface

A silent killer is stalking you, somebody you know, or somebody you love. Its name is hemochromatosis. It selects its victims mostly from among the young and productive, often maiming them or killing them at the peak of their careers.

We know the name of the killer and its modus operandi. We know how to recognize it early and take defensive measures. We know how to save the lives of its victims. All this we have known for half a century.

Nonetheless, this diagnosable, treatable disease continues to kill Americans and other nationals.

Part of the reason is lack of public awareness of hemochromatosis. Part of the reason is the persistence of three myths: (1) that hemochromatosis is rare and (2) that hemochromatosis is easily recognizable by history or physical examination or both, and (3) that the intestines block the absorption of any iron that is not needed.

Roberta Crawford has performed a very great public service in organizing Iron Overload Diseases Association. The organization has done much to alert physicians (and attorneys) to the dangers of hemochromatosis. *The Iron Elephant* will bring more public attention to the problems and hazards of hemochromatosis. The accounts she has given, of many actual cases, are each and all, medical horror stories: diagnoses made too late, proper treatment not given, needless suffering and tragic early deaths. Every case should have been diagnosed and treated early.

What can you learn from all this?

(1) The symptoms of hemochromatosis are extremely varied and may affect almost any organ of the body. They include fatigue, depression, arthritis, irregular heart beat, elevation in blood sugar, or diabetes, shortness of breath, swelling of the abdomen, swelling of the legs, jaundice, loss of sexual drive (impotence in men), pre-

mature menopause in women, loss of body hair, shriveling of testicles, hypothyroidism, and redness of the palms of the hands. An attractive suntan that does not fade in winter may come late or not at all in hemochromatosis. Your doctor may or may not find enlargement of liver, spleen, increase in blood glucose or in liver enzymes. If you have any of these symptoms or signs, you should be tested for hemochromatosis. But even if you do not have any of the above, you should be tested anyway, because these are late signs. It is far better not to wait.

(2) The test for hemochromatosis is simple and inexpensive. It is a test for serum iron concentration and the saturation, by iron, of its transport protein, transferrin.

Almost two thousand years ago, the Roman Pliny wrote: "the mischief that comes from iron is not the fault of iron, but of the unhappy wit of man."

Roberta Crawford's book may do much to remedy "the unhappy wit of man" as regards this stealthy killer.

—Virgil F. Fairbanks, MD
Department of Laboratory Medicine and Pathology
Mayo Clinic
Rochester, Minnesota

All of us, laypersons, physicians, scientists — know that a small amount of iron is needed for our bodies to function in a healthy manner. But few of us — laypersons, physicians, scientists — are aware that an excessive quantity of iron is a killer. Iron collects in our heart, our liver, our pancreas, our joints, and our pituitary gland. It accumulates and causes permanent heart damage, liver cirrhosis, cancers, diabetes, arthritis, gonadal decay, and damage to our infection defense system. Truly, the "iron heart" is not a strong heart — it has been pitifully weakened.

Among the few persons who are both knowledgeable about the dangers of iron overload and who have been alerting the public to the dangers is Roberta Crawford. Through the formation of Iron Overload Diseases Association, Inc., she has informed thousands of patients and many physicians about this very perilous yet very preventable and readily diagnosed condition. *The Iron Elephant* will alert hundreds of thousands. But even more remains to be done — in the United States alone, we have at least thirty-two million persons who carry the hemochromatosis gene!

We urge readers of *The Iron Elephant* to communicate its critical messages to members of their families, to their friends, and equally important, to their physicians. Our hope is that, by the year 2000, the concerted efforts of laypersons, physicians, and scientists will ensure that iron overload will no longer comprise one of the great plagues of humankind.

—Eugene D. Weinberg, PhD
Professor & Head Microbiology Section
Emeritus
Indiana University
Bloomington, Indiana

The Iron Elephant should be read not only by the public, but also by doctors and medical students. Incorrect views on iron are institutionalized not only in the medical profession, but also in industry and in government. Being read by lawyers, lawmakers and consumer advocates may also be needed to accomplish real change for the better. This book will save lives.

— Jerome L. Sullivan, MD, PhD
Clinical Assistant Professor Pathology
University of Florida
Gainesville Florida

Finally, with *The Iron Elephant,* we have the up-close-and-personal story of one of modern medicine's biggest oversights: the failure to diagnose iron overload, a potentially fatal and debilitating disorder. Roberta Crawford is uniquely qualified to spin this heart-wrenching, true-life tale of men, women and rust: She is the spokesperson for the thousands of sufferers who know and the millions who do not.

—Randall B. Lauffer, PhD
Assistant Professor
Harvard Medical School
Cambridge, Massachusetts

Roberta Crawford's tireless advocacy to increase early detection and adequate treatment has helped many individuals to avoid the ravages of untreated or unrecognized iron overload disease.The chapter headings of *The Iron Elephant* read like the outline for the postgraduate course in hemochromatosis. I applaud her continuing efforts to spread this important public health message.

—David L Witte, MD, PhD
Pathologist
Laboratory Control, Ltd.
Ottumwa, Iowa

The Iron Elephant is the most comprehensive, concise account of HH ever published. It's the best "refresher course" on HH I have had since I first started treating this illness in 1987. It is another reminder to treat this illness very aggressively.

The Iron Elephant will become "the bible" for patients, physicians and those interested in (iron overload diseases)." It is easy to read and succinctly reviews the history of HH, the clinical pictures, the "hurdles" in overcoming proper medical diagnosis and treatment: it also cogently emphasizes the need to insist on medical evaluation for iron overload, in the millions of North Americans who suffer from: chronic fatigue, abdominal pain, impotence, heart disease, diabetes and arthritis.

This book deservingly shakes up the medical community for their ignorance in and resistance to accepting HH as a common, disabling disorder.

When a doctor knows HH, he can help an additional twenty percent of his own practice and also truly practice preventive medicine.

—Paul Cutler, MD
Niagara Falls, New York

This trenchant and caring book's message - that diagnosis and prompt treatment of iron overload before damage is done pays off - is crucial for all: patients, their families, physicians, and health care systems.

—Sylvia S Bottomley, MD
Professor Medicine
University of Oklahoma College of Medicine
and Oklahoma City Veterans Affairs Medical Center

Roberta Crawford's sacrifices and dedicated efforts to write this second edition of *The Iron Elephant* are very enlightening and thought provoking. The results of this edition will be phenomenal in the prevention of very much miserable suffering and the saving of thousands of lives from too much iron. You will appreciate the extended and good life that you and your family will gain from what you learn from reading this book.

—Leslie N Johnston, DVM
Tulsa, Oklahoma

Acknowledgments

Many people have contributed in one way or another over the past twenty years to make this book possible. My special gratitude to Stephen Barfield, Alan Britt and Gene Allen for emotional support and for their insistence that I finish the manuscript, and to my father, Melvin Smith, who taught me that health is my own responsibility. Much gratitude to William H. Crosby, MD, for friendship and guidance and to physicians Walter G. Frey, III, Corwin Q. Edwards, Claus Niederau, Maria de Sousa, Herbert Bonkovsky, Victor Herbert, Lawrie Powell and James Barton, who are saving lives and teaching others.

I owe a great deal to Charles H. Brunie, R. Kevin Hackett, Louise Hyland, Joan Bergstrom, Dolores Forman, William Bacon and Sandra Ann Thomas for their unfailing support.

My gratitude to Robert W. Swisher, MD, who diagnosed my hemochromatosis and saved my life. He also made valuable suggestions on the text.

Others whose review and suggestions were enormously helpful are Virgil F. Fairbanks, MD; Sylvia Bottomley, MD; William D. Davis, Jr., MD; Eugene D. Weinberg, PhD; Jerome L. Sullivan, MD, PhD; Christopher F. Bryan, PhD and Randall B. Lauffer, PhD.

My sincere thanks to Rafael Tuburan for his help in copyediting. Peggy McQueen's assistance with computer problems was indispensable.

Recent valuable help has come from Vincent Felitti, MD; David Witte, MD, PhD; Ernest Beutler, MD; Paul Cutler, MD and Victor Gordeuk, MD.

Introduction

Isn't it ironic? We were told that lots of iron would make us strong. Isn't it ironic? How could everything they told us be so wrong? Now we supply the blood bank, slowing down the rust. Many of us are making frequent trips to the blood bank to unload excess iron that is rusting out our bodies and killing us.

The real irony is that most people carrying around this iron burden don't even know it. They never heard of iron overload. The medical term for the most common of the excess iron conditions is hemochromatosis.

This word is killing people. A word can actually kill? Yes. The word hemochromatosis conjures up in the mind of a typical physician a picture, a picture of an older man, bronze looking, with certain symptoms. Probably the man is already dying. I don't like a word that kills. I scorn a word that means only hemo (blood) chroma (with color) tosis (disease).

Iron overload is not a blood disease, and the patient's blood is not iron-rich. The excess iron gathers in the organs and tissue where it works its sinister injury. Iron overload is nothing but a condition of abnormal metabolism for iron, a metabolic defect.

And doesn't that word sound obscure? But it's much more common than you think. The excess iron oxidizes in your body and can "rust" out your liver, pancreas, joints, heart ... and places you don't want rusted out. You could get cirrhosis ... thrombosis ... arthritis .. impotence ... even cancer.

You might want to throw away those iron pills. The doctor prescribed them? Did he or she verify that your anemia is iron deficiency? With proper iron measures? If so, did he or she investigate to find the source of your internal bleeding or chronic infection or tumor? Should you pour iron down a sieve or feed bacteria or tumor cells? Or possibly parasites?

If iron is not that healthy additive we were all taught, why is it added to our foods?

Good question!

The Goal Of This Book

My goal in this book is to help us look at iron with new eyes. To help us see iron in a new light. We need to treat iron with respect for its potential for destruction. We have all been taught the wrong things about iron. We have been taught that it's difficult to get enough of it from our diet. It is embarrassing that too many in the medical community don't know the difference between hemoglobin and iron. Physicians were mistaught.

We were all taught that a low red blood cell count means iron deficiency and that if we are tired we may have "iron-poor blood." The media screams at us to pop iron. Selling iron to people who may be harmed by it is a "modern obscenity," according to physicians who are knowledgeable about iron. These physicians understand how to detect excess iron. They treat patients who are suffering the destructive effects of iron overload diseases. Scientists are studying iron's effects with increasing attention.

I had to learn these lessons in a hard and bitter way. Without knowing it, I was daily absorbing too much iron from food. At the same time doctors saw a pale, thin, *anemic* woman. Yes, anemic. The anemia resulted from B vitamin deficiencies, especially folic acid. Doctors in five American states gave me iron over many years. You can see that it was not just an occasional misguided physician who prescribed the iron, but several. Almost the entire medical community has until recently given exaggerated attention to anemia. The mild or borderline anemia would not have killed me, but the iron would have — and almost did.

Iron-loading anemia is much more common than physicians have been taught. Anemia is one symptom of iron overload! Unfortunately, doctors often fail to differentiate anemias. They too readily assume iron deficiency. Doctors have been unaware that some of their patients were dying because of a secret, silent overload of iron.

Luckily doctors are rapidly gaining awareness. Iron overload has become a hot medical subject.

Our new eyes need to see iron for what it is: a nutrient that is necessary for every body cell, but a deadly poison in excess. Virgil F. Fairbanks, MD, internist at Mayo Clinic, has reminded me that "Iron, after all, is one of the seven elements essential for life: carbon, oxygen, hydrogen, nitrogen, iron, phosphorous and sulphur." Dr. Fairbanks said, "Without iron we cannot even move a finger." Yes, you do have to have iron. However, getting enough of it is not the problem it has been made out to be.

Just try to design a reasonable diet that is iron-free. You can't do it. Iron is so abundant in food that it is impossible to formulate a sensible iron-free diet. Nutrition counselors have tried to devise diets without iron and found it impossible. Most people with iron overload are unaware, as I was, that their bodies are accumulating deadly iron stores. Those who have received a correct diagnosis hope to avoid iron, of course. They plead for a diet with low iron, but such a diet would lack other necessary nutrients. If you try eating only foods without iron, your diet will be bizarre indeed. There is no iron-free diet that is healthy.

There is enough iron in regular food to kill everybody. Why doesn't it? Most people are safe because their metabolism for iron protects them. A normal metabolism allows into the body the one milligram of iron daily that the body needs and can handle. A defective metabolism lets the body absorb too much.

It's true that only about ten percent of the iron in food is available for absorption. A good thing too. Once you absorb iron, it has no exit from the body except by blood loss. Unlike most other nutritional substances, iron is not excreted. Once allowed into the body, it takes up stubborn residence.

The red blood cell is born in the bone marrow and lives for about one hundred twenty days. When the red cell breaks down, it releases the iron, good as new, to be recycled into new cells. Only about one milligram a day is lost in finger nails, dead skin cells and other detritus, and this is the loss that needs to be made up from food.

You can see that since iron has no way of exiting, the delicate balance must be maintained through iron's entry into the body. Thank your normal metabolism for its ability to shut out excess iron; its ability to absorb only the amount needed. But what if your metabolism for iron is slightly defective? You may be able to get away with using iron additives for a certain length of time and your rejecting mechanism may work to protect you. However, some authorities believe that anyone can overwhelm his body with iron to the point of death. It is well known that a sudden tragedy can happen when a young child gets into his mother's iron pills. But this is different. I'm talking about slow, insidious poisoning from daily ingestion of additives and iron medication.

One day in 1978 a doctor said to me, "You have a rare and interesting disease, hemochromatosis." I had never heard the word. The doctor explained that it is a condition of excess iron stored in the body. I had never heard that it was possible for a human body to store too much iron. As a newspaperwoman, my first thought was to find out about it. I began researching this unheard of disorder. Today, more than two decades later, after numerous computer searches and intensive research, I still find the disease interesting, as the doctor said. Fascinating. Rare, however, it is not. We are learning that hemochromatosis is far from rare, is in fact common. Unfortunately, a correct diagnosis is still rare. A correct diagnosis followed by adequate treatment is rarer still.

Although iron overload is being increasingly diagnosed, treatment is still inadequate. Physicians seem afraid to take blood from their patients. The people I work with have learned what works and what does not. Timid treatment does not work. Diagnosis alone does not save the life.

The first time I was in a book store following that diagnosis, I picked up a copy of Stedman's Medical Dictionary Twenty-Third Edition, and turned to the horrible new word, hemochromatosis, to read, "a disease of older men." Older men? What about younger women? I sported no stubble on my chin. No hidden male parts. Older men! That definition was the first of a great many confusions and misconceptions I encountered in my search for correct information.

Later at the library my blood went icy when I read in "Trace Elements and Man" by Henry A. Schroeder, a description of hemochromatosis that concluded, "with death inevitable."

Most people have a normal iron metabolism that protects them from unneeded iron by rejecting the excess that's available in food. One theory says that a "mucosal block" operates a mechanism in the intestine that turns away excessive iron.

"Physicians, like other people, tend to act in accordance with their training and theories," writes Dr. Fairbanks. He writes, "There have been three widely taught, and widely accepted doctrines that have had a very deleterious effect on physicians' attitudes.

"1) The mucosal block theory, postulated in the late 1940s, and still widely believed by many physicians, holds that the intestinal mucosal cells will block the absorption of any iron that is not needed by the body. It has been because of this theory, that was based on the flimsiest evidence, that generations of physicians have believed that iron medication, when taken by mouth, cannot do any harm.

"2) The doctrine promoted by Dr. Richard MacDonald, of Boston, Massachusetts, that hemochromatosis is a non-entity, a figment of the imagination, and that it is really just alcoholic cirrhosis tinged with iron. This quite pernicious doctrine led many physicians not to worry about iron overload.

"3) The widely held belief that hemochromatosis is a rare disease and one that rarely affects women.

"Most physicians, I believe, try to follow the best information they have available, and these three doctrines are largely responsible for the reluctance of many physicians to accept the concepts that many of us have held for decades. We will succeed ultimately in changing these views ... I believe this is happening now, but it will not happen as quickly as we would like."

Much more needs to be learned about the "normal" iron range. Many people are secretly, unknowingly storing too much iron every day because, if there is a rejecting mechanism, it is missing or diminished. They are unable to keep from absorbing unneeded iron. Scientists estimate that one in two hundred people inherit this inability. Traditionally, recessively inherited diseases are rare because the affected individual has to inherit one gene from each parent to suffer full-blown effects. However, the single gene carrier rate is so high for iron metabolism defects that one out of every four hundred matings occurs between two carriers. Twenty-five percent of their children receive a double dose of the genes. French researchers report an estimated incidence of three in a thousand people with both genes and ten percent of the population with the single gene. Both Swedish investigators and University of Utah researchers are finding even higher prevalence: those scientists find one in two hundred people with both genes and one in eight carrying the single gene!

Some studies are finding even a much higher incidence. All of these figures are scientific estimates only. At present we know that the hemochromatosis gene is the most common abnormal disease-causing gene in America. We find this high prevalence everywhere in the world where iron has been measured. If we take the Utah figures — the middle of the road estimates — we see that more than one million Americans have the double H gene and that more than thirty-two million Americans are single gene carriers. That's well over a million and a half Americans and twenty-five million of the world's people. The single gene carrier estimate for the abnormality runs into six hundred fifty million people world-wide, more than a half billion. The most conservative estimate is that thirteen percent of the population does carry the single gene.

We are repeatedly told that iron deficiency is the most common nutritional problem in developing countries. Are true iron tests given to these people? If so, why are the tests more available in developing countries than in the U.S.? It is difficult for me to believe that multitudes of anemic people are being properly tested for iron levels. I say this because, in my experience, so many people are having a hard time to get their doctors to order iron testing, or even to interpret them correctly when they are done. Isn't iron deficiency the usual assumption made by doctors for all anemic patients? Iron deficiency is not a disease in itself, but a symptom. It can be a dietary problem or often in developing countries the result of parasites. Supplementing iron to nourish the parasites is not a logical solution. Many of the anemias may be caused by other nutritional deficiencies, or could be iron-loading themselves. Iron Overload Diseases Association (IOD) still receives too many reports from patients with thalassemia, an iron-loading anemia, who were treated with iron medication because their anemia was assumed to be iron deficiency! I have to conclude these mistaken assumptions are widespread.

If you are learning about iron overload here for the first time, you may be asking questions. Questions like: what does this iron overload do to you? I've never heard of it, so how common can it be? How in the world do you get it? Is it treatable? Can it be prevented? What are your chances of surviving if you have it? What kind of research is being done?

Perhaps you are skeptical. "This is just the opposite of everything I've always heard," you are saying. But you are speaking politely, and I thank you for that. Your mind is receptive to new knowledge.

"The Iron Elephant?" Many kinds of medical specialists are involved with various aspects of iron overload problems. Each doctor sees the subject from his or her own perspective like blind men describing an elephant. This dilemma was pointed out by Walter G. Frey III, MD, at a symposium in West Palm Beach, Florida. Dr. Frey displayed a cartoon of a large gray elephant surrounded by cardiologist, rheumatologist, gastroenterologist and others, each stationed at his point of interest. Dr. Frey referred to the story of the "Six Blind Men of Hindustan," who found the elephant "very like a rope;" or "very like a tree;" or "very like a wall," depending on the portion each was examining by touch.

The attempt here is to put together the widely separated parts of the elephant.

Instead of viewing iron overload as some special disease, look at the big picture. Everybody has iron. The question is: how much? When the amount is even a little too much, you need to give blood and get rid of the excess. Protect your good health .. and your life.

This book is going to answer your questions, and above all, this book is going to shine the bright light of new information on the subject of iron to help you see iron in a new light ... to look at iron with new eyes.

Roberta Crawford
North Palm Beach, Florida
January, 2000

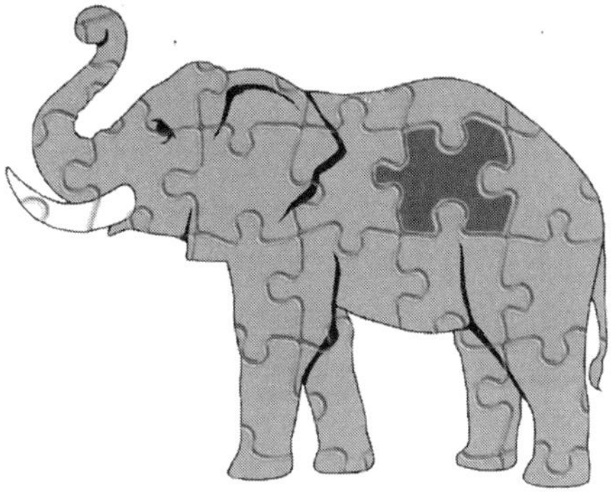

PART 1

"What would iron overload do to me?"

Chapter 1

Untreated Iron Overload Kills

The wedding date, May 6, 1984, was fast approaching. For months Rhonda's family had been busy working on plans to assure a lovely spring Alabama wedding. Rhonda radiated a rosy glow of happiness and excitement as she prepared for marriage to Alan, her high school sweetheart. As early spring buds began to appear and The Day came nearer, preparations intensified. So much still to be done! It would soon be May 6.

Rhonda died March 5th.

Iron overload was diagnosed on the autopsy table. Rhonda was twenty-three. Hemochromatosis is the medical name for the iron overload that killed Rhonda. The most common of the iron overload diseases, hemochromatosis dams body systems silently, secretly.

Hemochromatosis is fatal if not detected in time for adequate treatment. It's a wrongful death because a simple, effective treatment is available. Physicians look at their patients, fail to think of iron, fail to recognize the problem and allow their patients to die. Most patients do not receive autopsies, and most of these deaths join the iceberg of ignorance.

Rhonda had never taken iron supplements. She ate a normal

healthy diet. But each day her metabolic system accepted from food a little more iron than her body needed or could handle. The excess accumulated in storage organs and began slowly to injure them. Iron is one of the few nutrients that is not excreted. It remains in storage unless called upon to make replacement blood following hemorrhage. Blood loss is virtually iron's only exit from the body.

A strong warning had sounded, if anybody could have recognized it, when Rhonda was sixteen. That year, 1977, she told her mother she had stopped menstruating. Worse, she began suffering all the symptoms of menopause. No one understood why this was happening, but it was blamed on the strain of a strenuous school schedule.

Menstrual problems wave a red flag signaling that iron levels should be checked.

Friends found Rhonda's olive complexion and shapely body pretty, and she was fun to be with. All outward appearances reflected a happy, healthy teenager. No one thought to connect a year-round suntan with the possibility of accumulating iron.

By sixteen Rhonda had already made her career decision. She wanted to be an occupational therapist. Always busy, always active, she enjoyed doing volunteer work with emotionally disturbed children. She loved the children and it thrilled her when they responded to her friendship, when she could see them improving.

If you had known her then, you'd have responded too. She always had time for you, time to listen. One of her most unusual qualities was a delightful way of accepting people — anyone — without finding fault.

"So full of life," everybody said.

College stretched ahead and for Rhonda life was wonderful.

The Forman family enjoyed exceptional closeness. Dolores and Bob and their girls, Rhonda and Cynthia, spent just about every weekend on their houseboat at the lake, fishing, swimming, skiing, laughing. Alan joined them too, already like part of the family.

In early 1984 Dolores began cutting out her daughter's wedding gown, its white satin folds shimmering over the dining room table.

Rhonda, hectically busy, raced from classes at University of Alabama to volunteer work to wedding preparations. She was too joyous to give in to tiredness or joint pain. The slightest brushing against car doors left bruises. She had to force herself to meet deadlines and get everything done. But no matter, happiness radiated from Rhonda.

What a relief when finals were over and she could concentrate on the wedding. Now she had only to pass a national occupational therapy examination to get her license to practice. Her goals were clear to her. She took the exam and began waiting for the scores.

Her mother started sewing the gown and Rhonda stood for fittings. It wasn't easy. She became more tired; she started retaining fluid. Then she noticed a slight swelling of her whole body. Each day the fluid retention grew worse and finally the fluid began increasing her weight by six pounds a day. Dolores revised the dress daily. As she sewed, a worry started nagging at her. What could be wrong? Doctors had repeatedly insisted that laboratory tests revealed no abnormalities. Stress and overactivity, they said. Iron was not suspected; iron was not looked for; iron was not found.

Fatigue clamped down on Rhonda like a heavy blanket. Each effort became more of a struggle. Rhonda's heart was failing. Finally she confessed she couldn't go on without help, and her alarmed family got her admitted to a hospital.

That next week she grew steadily sicker. Her heart was damaged beyond repair, and doctors decided to prepare her for a heart transplant. Rhonda was still concerned about the results of the national occupational therapy examination for her license. Every day she asked, "Did the scores come?"

That week as Rhonda grew worse day by day, she began to know she would not get well. "They aren't going to diagnose me, mom," she said.

"I'm dying," she told Cynthia. The two sisters were close in age and close in affection. They had shared many a good time, many a laugh. "It'll be hard on mom and dad," Rhonda said. "You'll have to help them."

Rhonda remained alert until the moment her heart stopped.

That morning the test scores she had waited for arrived. Rhonda's marks were high.

Hemochromatosis is a condition caused by an abnormal metabolism for iron. The patient's metabolism allows more iron into the system than the body needs. Iron, unlike other nutrients, has no excretory pathway, no exit from the body. Instead, the excess must go into storage and the excess is laid down in organs and soft tissue where it works its damage. Where buildup is fast, the effects show up at an earlier age, and the heart takes the brunt of the damage, as in Rhonda's case.

Heart disease is usually the cause of death in young patients.

When stores accumulate slowly, the patient's heart is destroyed at a secret slower rate and he may keep living for decades to endure enough body damage to keep a dozen specialists busy.

Hemochromatosis can kill at any age from new born — even unborn — to 101.

When I began researching the condition in 1978 there was next to nothing in print for the general public. I was a newly diagnosed patient, and as with most patients, I craved information. In those days patients were supposed to keep their place and let doctors do the worrying. Medical librarians were likely to tell you that it was better for patients not to know too much. Medicine was filled with language understood only by doctors, and the codes were carefully guarded.

My son, Alan, got me into Johns Hopkins medical library with his alumnus card, and my journalism credentials helped elsewhere.

Thankfully this kind of nonsense has ended, and patients are now perceived as having the right to learn as much as they wish. In 1978 some medical texts omitted hemochromatosis, and there were dictionaries that referred to hemochromatosis as "a disease of older men." Others said it was "inevitably fatal." Despite the neglect of the subject in text books, much had been written in medical journals, as I found in medical libraries in Baltimore and at University of South Florida Medical School in Tampa. Gradually I learned enough to separate fact from chaff. I became able to pick out the authors in active research from those who were merely rewriting others' misconceptions.

I wanted to become active and work to help an organization that might be working for the disease. In 1978 I consulted Encyclopedia of Associations, but there was no such group listed.

My search of popular periodical indexes turned up not one article ever published in America on iron overload diseases. Magazines were however loaded with advice on iron deficiency.

I believe that part of the great general misconception about iron happened because, first, there was plenty of anemia. There was no way to measure iron before the 1950s, and all anemia was assumed to be caused by iron deficiency.

At that time I decided it was up to me to fill the gap, to start an organization and get information out to the medical community and to the public.

One of the most often quoted doctors writing about the disease was William H. Crosby. I located him, where he was working in the Distinguished Physician program at Walter Reed Army Institute of Research. He agreed by telephone to serve on our original Board of Directors. At that moment I felt we would eventually succeed in our goals. We outlined our mission as serving hemochromatosis patients and families and physicians, encouraging research and public information and pressing for earlier diagnosis and more effective treatment.

Even now, into a new Century, it is embarrassing that many physicians don't know the difference between hemoglobin and iron.

In 1980 I submitted an article to Good Housekeeping, whose editors of course consulted their medical advisers. Two doctors told them that the condition was too rare to bother with. However, a third doctor thought that hemochromatosis was increasingly emerging as a serious problem.

Good Housekeeping published "My Body Was Rusting Away," in November. About a hundred people tracked me down with calls and letters. Most told heart-tearing stories of family members killed by iron overload. They had died from delayed diagnosis and lack of adequate treatment. These survivors were bitter and sad. They cannot overcome the pain of knowing that death could have been avoided.

Others were themselves diagnosed, but only after much difficulty. Almost all of them had suffered irreparable damage and faced shortened lives.

It was clear that those scattered patients needed a place to turn. Most of them said they wanted to help keep others from suffering the misery they had known.

By then we began to recognize that most patients with hemochromatosis are dying without a correct diagnosis. It was clear that an organization was sorely needed. I had to feel my way cautiously, though. Questions, uncertainties, doubts besieged me. How could we, a small band of patients, see a picture that was invisible to so many doctors? I started traveling a thorny and slippery pathway through briars of misconceptions, searching for a clearing on solid ground. It was then that the invisibility of the problem turned into an iceberg. There but out of sight. Capable of inflicting destruction, but unseen. People dancing and singing above it and uninterested in hearing about it.

Walter G. Frey, Professor of Medicine at Dartmouth, was concerned that we might "scare people." I wrote to him that neither doctors nor patients were taking the condition seriously enough. Doctors were missing the diagnosis, and patients, even when diagnosed, did not understand the importance of adequate treatment. Maybe some fright was in order. Dr Frey agreed, and he joined our Board.

Right from the first the demand for information outstripped our shoestring budget. Patients were avid for information, and doctors also requested it. Many looked us in the eye and admitted they had "never heard of it." The media could not be convinced to give us space or air time. Commercials promoting iron additives or vitamins containing iron was a gigantic business. Funders answered our requests with form letters. How could this problem be as great as we claimed when no one ever heard of it?

By the late 1980s the Association, IOD, listed a world-wide membership of physicians, scientists and patients. IOD formed its official International Clearinghouse in 1985 — IOD-IC.

Charles sat on the side of his hospital bed at Miami's VA Hospital eating lunch. He was dying. He didn't know he was dying, but he knew that until years before that he had "never had a sick day." It was only two years earlier that symptoms began. It shows how silently iron works its destruction. And how fast and suddenly the body can collapse from the secret damage.

Now, though, Charles kept getting terrifying symptoms. The doctors only said he had something called hemochromatosis, the same as his brother in South Carolina.

I introduced myself that day — it was the Friday before Memorial Day Weekend — and explained to Charles that he and I had the same disease, and he told me his story.

Charles had been lounging with his wife at home in the Florida Keys one evening watching television when intestinal cramps seized him. That was not so unusual, but the black, tarry stool was. He opened a can of beer and said nothing to his wife, a nurse's aid.

In the night he got up vomiting blood, bowlsful of it. Now badly frightened, he meekly allowed Grace to call an ambulance.

That was in February. In the hospital his temperature shot to 104 and stayed there and doctors told him he had an enlarged liver. Also blood in his urine. The reason for that and the skipping heartbeat was unknown. At one point, he said, his blood pressure dropped to zero.

During Easter weekend he went home, but the black stools reappeared and Charles, in a panic, rushed back to the hospital. Now technicians had to transfuse him to replace the lost blood and keep him alive, and that was ironic. It was sad. Transfusion was the exact opposite of the treatment his disease required, if it had been discovered soon enough. He didn't understand all this.

In my own research I had learned that a sort of weeping from the portal vein of the liver into the abdominal cavity (ascites) is a manifestation of late stage disease.

There had been a warning two years earlier, but until then Charles had been more than unusually healthy. "Never a sick day," he told me. Many patients have a similar history of good health.

That first symptom had appeared two years before, when on Thanksgiving morning he had awakened with a high fever. He went to the local hospital in Tavernier, Florida. Doctors there couldn't identify the problem and he was transferred to the VA hospital, where hemochromatosis was also missed, but two years later, diagnosed.

His brother in Piedmont, South Carolina, was being treated for the same thing. But for Charles it was too late. He died a short time later.

The reasons for Charles' death, late diagnosis, and for Rhonda's death, lack of diagnosis, are recognized. However, most deaths that result from hemochromatosis are attributed to the immediate organ failure, and the excess iron is undetected. The cause of death may be listed as heart or liver failure, esophageal hemorrhage, diabetes or cancer. The underlying excess iron is more often than not, missed.

Hearing about the deaths of Rhonda and Charles along with many others that began pouring in spurred IOD to try everything we could think of to get the attention of the medical community and of the public to stop people from dying of this easily treatable condition. There was very little money, but we soon were working day and night.

In my innocence I thought all we had to do was let everybody know what was happening, and they'd be eager to fix it.

I was shocked that Rhonda died in 1984 after all our hard work since 1980.

Here it is now into a new century, twenty years later. Did the dying stop? Did it even let up? Our telephones are still drooping from new stories.

In February 1997 Tom Walsh Jr, a 37-year-old Southerner, died after a belated diagnosis the previous October. Liver cancer had already set in. His ferritin was 1700. Tom knew he was probably dying. He said more than once that at least he wanted his death to alert other people to know their iron level. He said, "Please tell people to test their iron and to have their loved ones tested."

A baby in Denver died after swallowing a number of iron pills. "Two thousand cases of iron poisoning occur every year in the U.

S. The Pink Sheet, published by FDC Reports, Inc., carried an item that American Association of Poison Control Center 'seeks label warnings and educational programs regarding accidental pediatric ingestion of iron-containing drug products or food supplements.'

"One-third of all accidental drug-related deaths among children under six were caused by iron tablets." [The Pink Sheet May 27 1991].

In November 1994 Agnes in Ishpeming Michigan said, "My 39-year-old son died. The doctor said the cause of death was iron overload." Then Agnes asked a question of the medical community. "Why does a person not know this before death?"

By the time Rhonda died and later when we learned of too many deaths to count, our message had been printed in a number of magazines and newspaper stories. We had been interviewed on every radio and television station that would take any interest. But our outreach had not touched Rhonda or Charles or Tom nor their physicians. Nor too many others.

A story by Mandy Matson in Parade Magazine and two columns by Ann Landers, who is widely circulated, actually led to diagnoses that people related to us. That cheered us and kept us going, but it's tough to overcome the frustration about the ones who still are being lost.

At the same time we are painfully aware that most people who have been killed by iron don't know it was iron that did it. Their families don't know it. Their physicians don't know it.

When iron overload has killed patients, in most cases, death is attributed to other causes. Even at autopsy iron will not be detected unless it is specifically sought.

The more layers we pull away from this disorder, the bigger we discover is the problem. I now call iron overload a national scandal, and it will remain so until the simple blood tests that measure iron are added to routine physicals.

You do not die when you discover the excess iron and remove it. Death occurs only when the iron is ignored or neglected. That fact makes this message urgent for everyone to know.

In 1996 Vincent Felitti MD, Director of Preventive medicine at Kaiser Permanente in San Diego, made a prediction. He said he was forced to predict that "a million Americans will die undiagnosed."

"Nobody in our country should die of iron overload," said David Witte MD PhD (Laboratory Control, Ottumwa Iowa) at a March 1997 meeting sponsored by the Centers for Disease Control. We had finally managed to get the CDC to take an interest. Traditionally the CDC has been more concerned with the kind of epidemics that come with infectious diseases. But Ray Yip MD became interested. Unfortunately he left soon after to work with UNICEF in Indonesia. The CDC invited many of the well known workers in iron overload to participate in that meeting.

If investigators don't suspect iron, they don't look for iron. If they don't look for iron, they don't find it.

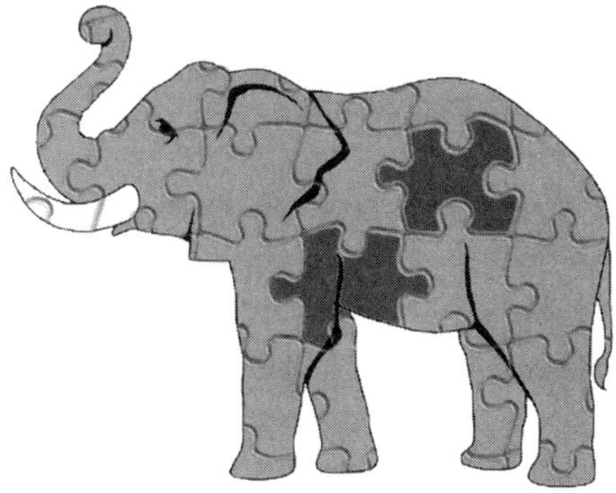

Chapter 2

Untreated Iron Overload Can Make You Impotent and/or Sterile

Jack worked for the United States Postal Service as a letter carrier in West Palm Beach. He walked and drove his route during steamy Florida summers under a blazing sun and during mild winters. In the 1960s his health began deteriorating steadily. Jack forced himself to keep going despite a cycle of influenza infections with high fevers and severe headaches. He sought help from physicians but relief eluded him. The constant illnesses were confusing enough, but what depressed him most was a failing libido. "It's because I'm so tired," he told himself.

Lessening sexual desire can be an unwelcome early warning of iron overload. The lover who finds himself in that awkward position may very well save both his potency and his life by demanding proper testing of his iron levels.

As disease progresses, the iron destroys pituitary function and causes shriveling of testicles. In women excess iron may lead to atrophy of the ovaries. IOD conducted a survey in 1984. Results show that a high proportion of female patients have undergone hysterectomy, possibly as a result of their physicians' practice of treating symptoms instead of looking for causes; possibly because hypopituitarism, a condition of deficiency of the pituitary gland, can be an early development of iron overload.

A doctor told Jack he had picked up a "rare jungle disease" while fighting in World War II. His legs took on a strange black and blue color. "Dermatitis," said another doctor. Jack became completely impotent. In desperation he went to doctor after doctor — a common experience of iron overloaded patients. He went to the Cleveland Clinic. He went to a Veterans Administration hospital in Michigan. That's where the diagnosis was finally made.

"I'm sorry ... if we had seen you earlier."

Iron overload was detected three months before death.

Impotence is one of the inconveniences — many would say tragedies — of hemochromatosis. And some authorities say no improvement can be expected even with treatment once damage has taken place. Iron buildup damages the anterior pituitary and adrenal glands, and that damage leads to insufficiency of the gonad. The gonad is the primary sex gland, which depends upon the pituitary and adrenal secretions for hormone production. In men the gonad is the testicle; in women it is the ovary. The iron damage reduces the production of male or female sex hormones, testosterone in men, estrogen in women. This reduction decreases libido and eventually sometimes causes testicular atrophy and loss of sex function or cessation of menses.

With hemochromatosis, pituitary and adrenal glands become pigmented and scarred in many cases. Yet each individual has a unique metabolism and the degree of damage varies. Improvement after treatment has been demonstrated, however, in some studies.

A young woman wrote a newsletter for IOD in 1989 telling her story. Jennifer said, "I should have been diagnosed at age 11 when tests showed high iron and elevated liver enzymes." Amazing and unusual that these tests were made. But what good are tests if you are going to ignore the results?

Jennifer said that "hemochromatosis was mentioned on my chart. Unfortunately the doctor did not follow up. He was satisfied to call it hepatitis." IOD has heard this same comment over and over. The physician writes "hemochromatosis" on the chart followed by a question mark. I want to point out that if such a possibility crosses your mind, you dare not fail to investigate in view of the consequences.

Jennifer continues. "The delay of 15 more years has caused me an immeasurable amount of heartache and pain. I was always one of the more athletic children in my neighborhood until the 'hepatitis.'

Over the next 15 years my endurance steadily declined. I couldn't understand why I had turned into such a 'lemon.' Diets, exercise, nothing worked. I was always exhausted."

This confusion and guilt are repeatedly spoken of as an early feature of iron loading.

Jennifer said that at the age of 24 something happened that she couldn't figure out. Her periods stopped. The same thing had happened to her sister at age 28. Her sister had also undergone years of declining health and had developed diabetes. Her color took on a greenish tone, causing worry to the family. Finally Jennifer's sister was diagnosed. A physician had measured her transferrin saturation and serum ferritin. At last! The rest of the family was then tested. That included Jennifer, who now had some answers. Her ferritin was 4800.

At first phlebotomies were hard for her. Then she says she started thinking of the iron as poison. She became motivated to unload the toxic iron as fast as possible and made a schedule of two phlebotomies a week. To do that she had to give up a glamorous job in Hollywood and moved back home with her mom in Florida.

Just before she left Los Angeles Jennifer met another patient who was as despairing as Jennifer felt at that time. Jill, a teacher, was on a phlebotomy program of one every other month. Of course she was going downhill. Timid treatment does not work. Only vigorous treatment works. Jennifer convinced Jill to treat her disease aggressively, and Jill had to quit working and move in with her brother.

"But here's the best part," says Jennifer. Her periods resumed. Now she again thought of her dream of having a baby. Jill kept in touch by phone and reported that she is well again too. Now healthy she feels she has a bright future.

Jennifer is back exercising again, held a full-time job in New York and felt "very lucky." She says, "I know that most people never receive a correct diagnosis."

But here's the real best part. After Jennifer's iron was all cleared out she married and gave birth to a wonderful baby boy. That reversal of sterility didn't happen because of diagnosis. It happened because of correct vigorous treatment.

Rhonda was struck down at twenty-three. Charles and Jack both died in their fifties. Rhonda and Charles were relatively well until end stage, but Jack suffered prolonged illnesses. These differences show how variably iron overload expresses its power.

When you consult a professional about any kind of sexual or reproductive dysfunction, you are not receiving proper help if your iron status is ignored. Iron overload is the single most often neglected cause of sexual impotence and sterility. Your sexuality problems are not being thoroughly investigated unless therapists measure your iron levels.

A Wisconsin businessman kept suffering a bewildering series of ailments. He went to doctors who gave him "every medical test in the book." Unfortunately doctors failed to order iron tests. The oversight cost Gerald his health and forced him to sell his business. A bitter consequence of the excess iron was loss of sexual potency.

Gerald learned of IOD and became a member. He began collecting information on his medical problems. Later he said he just could not understand how doctors missed his diagnosis. As a layman, he said, "If I had had access to the information back then, I could have diagnosed myself."

Often the patient will notice loss of body hair, resulting from the iron deposits in the pituitary gland. Women sometimes experience cessation of menstruation. We also hear from women who report an abnormally heavy menstrual flow. More than one of these women have speculated, "Could this have been my body's attempt to get rid of the iron?"

Can you imagine the grief of knowing that you had lost your husband, daughter, mother to a disease that is easy to detect and easy to treat?

The sad stories that poured into IOD offices in the early years kept volunteer workers in a subdued if determined frame of mind, with very little humorous relief. One day though the tension broke after we re-read a letter we wrote to a young Australian woman. Her father had died of hemochromatosis. The woman herself suffered symptoms, and she had written to IOD for counseling. She said she was unable to get pregnant. Could we help her?

"Visit Dr. Lawrie Powell in Brisbane," we wrote. "We believe he can get you pregnant."

It struck us funny on the re-reading, which shows you how hard up we were for a good laugh.

Many months later we met Dr. Powell, and that eminent authority on hemochromatosis smiled tolerantly at our little story.

Any experience with lessening libido or change with menses or difficulty conceiving should motivate you first to check iron levels. Getting rid of excess iron before it grows to Titanic proportion could save you much grief as well as money.

Better yet, don't wait for such injury. If you bother to know how much you weigh or if you keep track of your blood pressure, do the same with ferritin and percentage of saturation. Set a limit on how high you'll allow ferritin to rise. (Six is good.) Become a blood donor and keep extra iron cleared out.

The old myth that iron deficiency was at the root of low sexuality was dead wrong. Iron itself is strong enough, but in excess it confers no strength or energy or sexual benefits on the human body. You may remember the Geritol commercials in the old days of television. A sexy woman revealed that she took Geritol daily because it contained more iron than calves liver. Then her husband, with a horny leer would say, "My wife, I think I'll keep her." Then he would add, "And she makes me take it too."

After it became better known that males certainly do have plenty of iron, the ads dropped that part of the story. But anemic females were so well entrenched in popular belief that the drug companies continued to advise women relentlessly to use their dangerous concoction. All the while they ecstatically raked in enormous stacks of the drug money. Knowledgeable physicians filed complaints. As Walter G Frey III MD said to me one day, "TV hucksterism to sell iron to those who don't need it is a modern obscenity."

The Federal Trade Commission (FTC) revealed a considerable impotence itself in dealing with this disgraceful situation. The mammoth ad campaign was illegal in the first place. It was illegal to mislead the public into believing that all fatigue and low sexual desire was caused by "iron-poor blood." A campaign of hearings took place and the FTC told the advertisers to "cease and desist." However advertising continued with only a few changes, and the FTC contented itself with feeble protests.

Geritol profited by piggy-backing on the oft quoted myth that iron deficiency is the world's most common nutritional problem. The US Government made the same error that many physicians are still making: that hemoglobin measures iron.

Jerome L Sullivan MD PhD says, "Incorrect views on iron are institutionalized not only in the medical profession, but also in industry and in government."

Geritol continues being sold and continues being advertised with its misleading claims.

Among those who may not need iron are pregnant women. A paper concerning the standard practice of routinely prescribing iron in pregnancy appeared in JAMA. The writer advised testing the woman's hemoglobin to determine iron status before medicating!

Victor Herbert MD JD warns that legal action may follow if iron is given without testing iron levels.

A physician on the internet wrote, "Doctors get into habits that are hard to break." He claims he never gives iron to a pregnant woman unless he has proven that she needs it. Let's add to that, does she know her metabolism for iron? Does she know the baby's metabolism? Is she eating food?

Testing may not tell the full story. A 1997 study reported that 6.2 percent of 65 women tested with normal saturation and ferritin though severe disease was present in some. None of the 30 men tested normal. All were homozygotes for hemochromatosis, based on HLA.The study concluded that menstruation and pregnancy do not exclude women from iron overload.

Since the popular pharmaceutical product, Viagra (Sildenafil) became available, a male might decide just to fall back on that fix rather than finding a cause for his failing libido.

But keep in mind that there is more than sex to be lost if your body is playing host to a growing supply of iron.

Most people whose impotence or sterility is iron caused, are unaware they have iron overload.

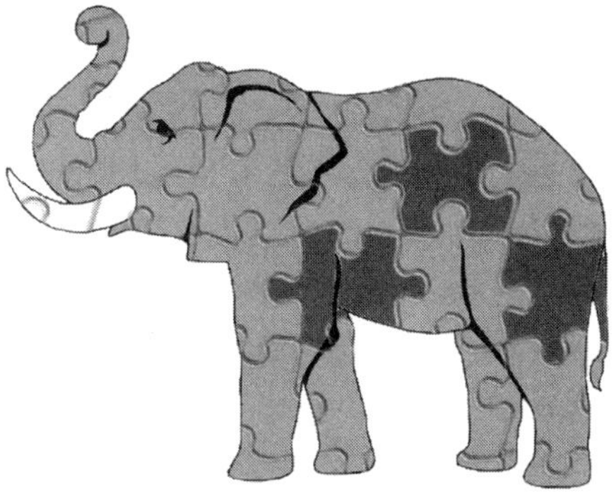

Chapter 3

Untreated Iron Overload Can Give You Cancer

Robert was a five-foot eleven inch, 130- pound father of five sons and a daughter, a much loved family man. The family lives near Detroit. After Robert gave up smoking in the 1960s he began putting on weight, up to about 160. The thirty extra pounds were noticeable on a man who had been thin.

Ten years later in 1975 Robert received a diagnosis of diabetes, and his weight dropped back to 130. He turned out to be a "brittle" diabetic. Sugar levels flared out of control. A few times he went into insulin shock. A consulting physician penciled a note on his medical record: hemochromatosis? That suspicion was not followed up, tragically. Any time diabetes appears, such a diagnosis ought to emit a screeching blast of warning: CHECK IRON.

Robert's daughter, Suzanne, is an artist, mostly in fiber sculptures. She says that her father was put into the hands of an endocrinologist, a specialist in diabetes. She says the doctor was looking at his patient from his own one narrow viewpoint. At IOD we call it seeing only one small part of the elephant.

Robert kept working until 1982 when he became so ill he had to take early medical retirement. Suzanne called his doctor. "Well, his numbers look fine," the doctor said. If he had checked Robert's iron levels he would have seen numbers that were not fine.

It took nine years from the diabetes diagnosis before Robert's excess iron was detected. When he was hospitalized for a heart condition, hemochromatosis was not suspected because he did not fit the picture in the minds of his doctors. Robert's skin was too fair with no bronzing.

Robert died of liver failure in the intermediate care unit of a Michigan hospital. He had developed cancer of the liver. During his remaining seven weeks of life, Robert's medical bills mounted to over a hundred thousand dollars.

Excessive storage iron in the liver is carcinogenic for primary liver cancer. Studies show that a third of all diagnosed patients develop cancer, if the diagnosis is made after sufficient damage to cause cirrhosis (scarring of the liver). Liver cancer has been found to be 219 times more frequent among hemochromatosis patients who were diagnosed after cirrhosis had developed or whose iron burden was too great to be removed within eighteen months (NEJM 1985;313:1256-62). If cirrhosis has not yet developed, and treatment is adequate, liver cancer rarely develops.

It had long been known that the cancers occurred even after all excess iron was removed. Some workers believed the tumors resulted from irreversible organ damage. This was shown to be so from the German study mentioned in the New England Journal of Medicine report cited. The report electrified researchers around the world by revealing that early detection — before cirrhosis — and prompt removal of excess iron — within eighteen months — permits the individual to live out a normal life span in normal health. Such early detection also appears to prevent the later development of liver cancer.

By the time Robert's iron overload was finally recognized, a mass was already growing in his liver. Robert gave blood biweekly and later monthly. (Timid treatment). When the tumor grew malignant Robert made the decision for surgery. Surgeons removed the left lobe and part of the right, seventy percent of the liver.

Suzanne now feels that if her father had foreseen the pain and "humiliation" a patient endures in intensive care, he would not have elected the surgery. During the last days his family stayed with him constantly. Their deep frustration lingers. It's the knowing that he could be with them today to enjoy holidays with them if doctors had made a correct diagnosis years earlier. We should say if doctors had made the correct diagnosis and then had followed up with intensive treatment.

A link between excess iron and leukemia was reported in June Goodfield's thrilling book, An Imagined World, a record of scientific discovery." (Harper & Row, Penguin Books). This true story details the work of a young Portuguese scientist delving into the mysteries of the immune response system. The scientist was studying immunology, not iron. At the very beginning of her career in London, "Anna" (the pseudonym used for the scientist) stared through the lenses of her microscope and experienced a moment of illumination, a flash of insight.

Anna made the astonishing discovery that each of the two lymphocyte populations, known as the T cells and the B cells, occupies its own separate area. In the quiet exhilaration of exploring scientific frontiers, Anna pursued the secret leucocytes. Could it be, she speculated, that, contrary to all accepted belief, could it be that in Hodgkin's disease, for example, or leprosy, the leucocytes are not diminished, but are simply trapped in areas other than where they belong?

Her speculations proved correct — and iron proved to be the trapping agent. When evidence became incontrovertible, the scientist began publishing her work. Her first paper was presented to a silent and stunned audience of her peers at a meeting of the British Society of Immunologists, and was published in the Journal of Experimental Medicine.

More surprises! In leukemia, does iron inhibit cell differentiation in the bone marrow? This link is still in the process of being investigated.

Meanwhile we have learned that iron does depress the immune system. Tumors require iron. For this reason when there is a finding of iron deficiency, you must search for cancer. You must consider the possibility that iron is being gobbled up by the tumor and therefore is not available for blood formation. A good reason not to medicate with iron, even in iron deficiency.

Anna knew right away her discovery would not be popular. It upset too many rigidly held misconceptions about the place of iron in the human body.

IOD is now uncovering families where both hemochromatosis and leukemia are present. Both conditions are common enough to occur together by coincidence. Yet a strange resistance to new perspectives persists. A relationship of iron overload and cancer is becoming clear. The can of worms is open; facts are wriggling to freedom. Painful as it may be for us to admit our past ignorance, now we have to be receptive to new knowledge. The problem is, there is a certain amount of vested interest in clinging to outworn "facts." Authorities who previously published such "facts" and put their names to advice they gave in all sincerity — advice that conformed to general beliefs of the time — may find it impossible to reverse themselves. Understandable. Others are in the pay of food or drug companies as consultants. Their sincerity may be colored, tinted, tainted by bills to be paid. And what can we say to physicians, good doctors, who are now being told they buried patients from whom they should have been removing iron instead of adding to the iron overload? Rigidly held beliefs that are not exposed to continuing investigation have no place in science or art or medicine.

We must be willing to learn.

"The anti-cancer drugs developed in the last two decades are almost as lethal as the diseases they are intended to defeat," writes Diane B. Paul in the New York Academy of Sciences publication, Science in Focus Vol 1 No. 3. "It is known that they don't work well in the long run and have unpleasant, sometimes disastrous side effects."

Cancer cures are waiting for the future. It appears our best defense is still prevention.

Sometime during our new Century when we have convinced people to know their ferritin levels — and then to keep them low by blood donations — we'll see a rejuvenation of people's health. Money now being misspent on medical problems will be available for other luxuries as well.

Robert's liver cancer was a direct result of his undiagnosed and timidly treated iron overload. He had seven sisters and one brother, and all but two have been diagnosed with iron overload. Robert's diagnosis saved the lives of his sisters, who are being treated. The eldest, however, is anemic and should have but did not receive phlebotomies.

Eugene D. Weinberg, PhD, has conducted studies at Indiana University on the relationship of cancer to iron. Writing in Biological Trace Element Research 3, 55-80 (1981) he quotes a study that found that "in twenty humans, the mean dry weight of iron in breast cancers was threefold greater than that of normal breast tissue." (P.M. Santoliquido, H. W. Southwick and J. H. Olwin, Surg. Gyn. Obstet. 142,65 (1976). It has been found that eighty-eight percent of patients with metastasizing breast cancer had elevated serum ferritin (storage iron) levels. (R.C. Coombs, T. J. Poules and J. C. Gazet, Cancer 40, 937 (1977).

In Hodgkin's disease Maria de Sousa, MD, PhD, proposed that the central defect is a failure of the spleen and lymph node macrophages to handle iron normally. For a period of years de Sousa had been working on the iron-cancer link at Sloan-Kettering Cancer Institute and later at Harvard Medical School.

Weinberg demonstrated that in both infection and malignancy iron is shifted to storage tissues. The severity of cancer is related to displacement of iron. Moreover, when the patient recovers, the iron levels return to normal.

This is why it is essential to investigate for cancer or infection when transferrin saturation or serum ferritin test low. Internal bleeding will also cause low iron measurements. The individual who takes iron just because his blood work shows low iron levels is turning off the fire alarm and ignoring the fire.

Your body attempts to withhold iron from tumor cells, and can do this more successfully when you are not iron overloaded.

Weinberg observed that a number of cases of sarcoma have developed at the site of injection of iron dextran.

Inhalation can be another mode of entry for iron. Workers in iron mines developed bronchial cancer five to ten times the rate of the general population. Although questions were raised about the purity of the studies regarding iron workers, the same thing happened to hamsters, who, though, not forced to work in mines, were forced to inhale iron oxide. The hamsters did develop neoplasms in the lower respiratory tract.

Tobacco is another source of iron. The plant is iron-rich, and smokers add the mineral directly into their lungs. Weinberg concludes that animals and humans "burdened with excess iron appear to have a greater than normal risk of developing one or more primary neoplasms."

Most iron-related cancers are hepatomas, that is, liver cancer. However many studies report a variety of tumors. A Swiss study shows that lung cancer was 7.5 times higher than expected in patients with hemochromatosis. Other cancers recorded were pancreas, stomach, rectum, gallbladder and brain.

The writers, R. W. Ammann, E. Muller, J. Bansky, G. Schuler and W. H. Hacki related another study in which cancers were found in bladder, colon, ileum and prostate.

Hepatomas tend to occur when there is long-term irritation of the liver cells. The irritation can come from virus, alcohol - or iron. Once the irritation causes scarring (cirrhosis) there is the potential for a malignant tumor to appear.

Liver cancer is now the most common cause of death in hemochromatosis patients, even among those treated. Vigor of treatment does make a difference.

At risk individuals should be screened annually with alpha feto protein (AFP). The numbers should be below 50. High levels are found in at least 70 percent of patients who develop this hepatoma. AFP can give indications of other cancers as well: testes, ovaries, pineal gland or gastrointestinal tract.

Maria de Sousa with Daniel Potaznik, produced a paper for "Vitamins, Nutrition and Cancer," pp 231-239 (Harger, Basel 1984). The question they considered was: In countries with adequate iron intake, where the incidence of bacterial infection is low, do malignant cells that develop effective mechanisms of iron uptake have a survival advantage?

In a study of twenty-two children with leukemia, iron levels were measured. Five of the children with the most severe disease suffered relapses. Transferrin saturation (a measure of iron levels) of the five were recorded at 23%, 86%,91%, 50% and 100%. Only the child with the 23% of transferrin saturation survived.

De Sousa concluded with an answer to her posed question:

"hosts with high serum iron, high transferrin saturation and high serum ferritin may provide a more favorable environment for neoplastic growth."

In summary de Sousa noted "the increasing incidence of cancer in countries with low incidence of bacterial infection in which iron fortification programs have been implemented."

"Thus," concluded de Sousa, "the iron store status of the host can be a critical determining ecological influence on neoplastic growth."

In February, 1994 Science News quoted Lawrence A Loeb of the University of Washington in Seattle as saying,"If iron is really a carcinogen, we're facing a lot of debate." He mentioned that a Food and Drug Administration regulation prohibits the adding of carcinogens to food.

William H Crosby MD had been saying the same thing for years. In Nutrition Today (July/August 1986) he said, "The Delaney Amendment ... prohibits the addition of carcinogens to food. Although iron is naturally present in all foods, it is well known as a carcinogen." Crosby pointed out that "The addition of iron to food is illegal."

Cancer Research in 1988 published a study that described decreased tumor growth in iron-deficient mice. Two groups of mice, fifteen in each group, were studied. Group One were fed a low iron diet and Group Two were fed normal iron. All the mice were inoculated with tumor cells, colon, liver and breast tumors.

At each observation the largest tumors were in the normal iron group. Tumor growth in the iron-deficient group continued to be significantly slower, and tumors remained smaller. Metastasis was seen in six of the normal iron group and in only one of the low iron group.

Authors of the study said that "Iron is known to be an essential element for growth of all cells including tumor cells." They suggested that "iron supplementation in cancer patients or older people at high risk of cancer might enhance tumor growth." They said "This knowledge should be considered when designing treatment for patients with cancer. Iron oversupply in cancer patients might enhance tumor growth and adversely affect cancer therapy." [Hie-

Won L. Hann, Mark W Stahlhut and Baruch S Blumberg]. In a similar study published a year later [Int. J. Cancer: 43, 376-379] Hann was able to make the suggestion that "Therapeutically, use of chelating agents (deferoxamine) or phlebotomy might be considered as methods to decrease total body iron stores."

Let's add to that suggestion that if the cancer has not already made the patient iron deficient, let's go ahead and reduce the iron burden. And before cancer appears let's remove all excess iron, taking the ferritin to below ten, and deny the essential iron to any opportunistic cancer cells.

Richard G. Stevens produced a study in 1988 from the Pacific Northwest Laboratory in Richmond, WA. Stevens' study of 14,000 healthy Americans found that men with high iron levels were 37 percent more likely to develop cancer than those with low levels. Stevens said that individuals should give blood to reduce cancer risk. Add this proposal to your cancer prevention plan.

Another 1988 study at Fox Chase Cancer Center in Philadelphia found that early cancer could be detected in 92.3 percent of cases by using a measurement of a combination of serum ferritin and alpha feto protein. The malignancies most closely associated with elevated ferritin were liver, breast, lung, leukemia, Hodgkin's lymphoma, multiple myeloma and neuroblastoma.

Weinberg wrote in 1991 that "hosts might be able to restrict neoplastic cell growth by withholding or withdrawing iron from the malignant cells." He mentioned that numerous reports have been published that cancer patients who receive excessive transfusions of whole blood often see accelerated tumor recurrence and decreased survival. Weinberg said this was usually explained as caused by unknown allogeneic antigens, while "oddly, the potential role of iron ... has not been considered." It's the iron!

"Iron can destroy anything: families, fortunes, governments, whole countries. It's the most powerful stuff in the universe," wrote John Jakes in North and South. Jakes was speaking of weapons of war. But the same mineral is every bit as destructive when it accumulates excessively in a human body.

During the 1990s crime was a serious issue in everybody's mind. The murder rate was one in 10,000 annually. The hemochromatosis one-time rate is 50 times that! Iron accumulating inside the human body is every bit as deadly as the lead in bullets.

A letter to the editor in The Miami Herald spoke of her grief over her father's death. She wrote, "One can be sure that if a serial killer were stalking and killing 12 people a year in Florida, information, investigation, publicity and warning would be abundant! But not for a smoking gun in the form of raw oysters! How many people are going to die or be irrevocably poisoned into a life of neuromotor deficiency because ... no one cares?" Her father had died after eating raw oysters. This happens when the individual has undiagnosed iron overload. The excess iron feeds a common bacterium that appears in raw seafood. The same food is harmless to those without the excess iron to provide food for the bacteria. More about this later.

Bacteria and cancer cells cannot live without iron.

Remove excess iron before it injures key organs, and your risk of cancer becomes the same as that of the general population.

Most people who die of iron-caused cancer never knew — and their doctors are unaware — that iron overload was the deciding factor in their failure to survive.

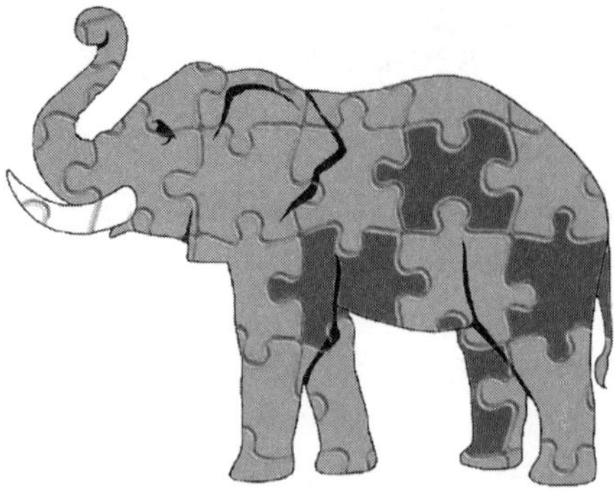

Chapter 4

Untreated Iron Overload Can Give You Arthritis

A photo of Rhonda taken a few months before death shows a slight crookedness of her fingers. Arthritis is virtually a universal symptom of fully developed hemochromatosis. You may first notice sore or stiff fingers. Specific parts of the hands may be affected, index and middle finger, for example. This is the most typical arthritis of hemochromatosis. However, hand pain and body pain can vary. It may depend upon overuse or straining. If someone shakes your hand with a hurting grip and the pain lingers, you should arrange to test your iron levels.

Other joints become sore or aching, inflamed or swollen: knees, hips, jaw, shoulder.

Donald is a California dentist. He is outraged that he suffers permanent disability because his arthritis was misdiagnosed as rheumatoid arthritis. Treatment for rheumatoid arthritis is useless when the patient's arthritis is iron caused. Donald wasted years and accumulated huge medical bills undergoing treatment that proved ineffective. He faithfully followed the advice of his specialist, a noted rheumatologist.

Finally Donald submitted to a hip replacement. Numerous complications of iron overload began appearing, and ultimately overwhelmed him. The dentist, still young, has bitterly retired from practice.

Joint pain is not always present. It is not a necessary feature of hemochromatosis. Some studies show that only fifty percent of patients suffer arthritis. But arthritis is a strange malady that has a tendency to come and go. Patients who contact IOD almost always report joint involvement unless their diagnosis was made in the earliest stages.

Betsy, a New York City executive, had been treated for arthritis over a period of thirteen years. One day a doctor noticed tiny red specks on Betsy's legs. She ordered a serum ferritin test, which measured 2400. Normal for women is usually less than 200. Betsy is grateful for the diagnosis. "I only regret," she says, "that my arthritis doctor, now retired, didn't spot the iron overload fifteen years ago. I thought the lowered energy was part of growing older." Betsy was fifty.

The joints most often affected are those of the hands and wrists, as well as weight-bearing joints such as knees. Rheumatologists should be alert for periarticular rarefaction, narrowing and cystic changes of the second and third metacarpal heads. A phenomenon sometimes seen is Dupuytren's contracture, a condition of the palm that can interfere with finger movement and even in severe cases, contract the hand into a claw. However, this is not in any way specific for iron overload.

A small portion of skin is bound to connective tissue, preventing free movement. When something similar happens in other parts of the body — cheeks, stomach, arm — it is called panniculitis. The flesh seems to fasten to connective tissue. It can be a tiny dimple or a larger depression.

Charles' brother, J. T., underwent surgery for Dupuytren's contracture, but the operation succeeded only in opening the fingers and J. T. lost the use of his hand.

Along with polyarthritis there may be acute synovitis, an inflammation of the membrane that sheaths tendons. The most common kind of iron-caused arthritis is chondrocalcinosis, also known as pseudo-gout, caused by iron deposits in the joints or by iron injury to the joints. The mechanism is not understood.

Maria de Sousa, MD, PhD, writing from Harvard Medical School, said that "The mechanism by which iron contributes to synovitis may relate to stimulation of the formation of toxic oxygen radicals..." She said, "Exacerbation of synovitis has been reported in (rheumatoid arthritis) patients receiving iron dextran infusions for anemia."

IOD hears more comments about the struggle to live with arthritis than any other of the many injuries brought about by iron. Arthritis is also one of the most difficult symptoms to improve.

National Arthritis News, Vol. 3, printed remarks from studies conducted by David R. Blake, MD and Paul A. Bacon, MD, working at University of Birmingham in England. "We suggest that iron may directly affect rheumatoid inflammation and advise precaution in its prescription to those with early disease." The researchers said that "iron promotes the growth of bacteria, which can contribute to the inflammation associated with arthritis."

William G. Benson and his colleagues wrote a case report in which they commented, "It is important to distinguish hemochromatosis arthropathy from other arthritic diseases both to avoid unwarranted therapy and to allow early treatment with phlebotomy." *(Arthritis and Rheumatism,* Vol. 21, No. 7 1978). They said, "Some authors suggest that phlebotomy improves survival and may prevent or reverse some of the clinical manifestations..." and "Although arthritis is not affected by phlebotomy and may occur after iron stores are depleted, its recognition may allow early diagnosis and treatment ... Furthermore, potentially toxic drugs or surgical therapy for other rheumatic diseases may be avoided."

Hip replacement has become so common among iron overloaded patients, that the necessity for the procedure is almost as good as a test for iron. Many other orthopedic surgeries are submitted to by patients, as well. The expense and pain of all this can very often be prevented if the patient's iron level is lowered soon enough and kept low. Hemochromatosis is an interesting disease from a medical viewpoint, but what it does to you is hideous. Your organs and tissues become fibrous, scarred, shriveled and pigmented a brownish or rusty color. How ugly they must be and how lucky you are that they are undercover of the body's skin. Secretly knowing the condition of your inner body you feel grateful to have your skin wrapping and enclosing it all out of sight.

But of course the skin, too may become pigmented and atrophied.

While being treated for hemochromatosis you can usually go

ahead with normal living. One day you are out with your husband on the way to a nice place for lunch. You're discussing his new Mozart album and what to do about the stereo and will a hurricane come this season. At your vision's edge a sinister view tugs at your attention. High wooden walls vainly try to contain the ugliness of a junk yard. You avert your gaze, but not quickly enough to avoid the sudden spectacle of unsightly rusted out automobiles. The obscenity of exposed ruined bodies, eaten through by oxidized iron rust. Once they were so dazzling and expensive, so prized, now abandoned for junk. Iron rust in a human body is not the same as iron rust in a Detroit product. Still it does take a mental adjustment to disentangle yourself. Before rusting you out beyond salvage, hemochromatosis invades the vital organs, building slowly but inexorably. It presents a mysterious symptom here and a puzzling one there. You'll need an unusually alert physician to recognize these symptoms. They will not be the same in all patients. Virtually every symptom can also indicate an entirely different condition.

Most people whose arthritis is iron caused are unaware they have iron overload.

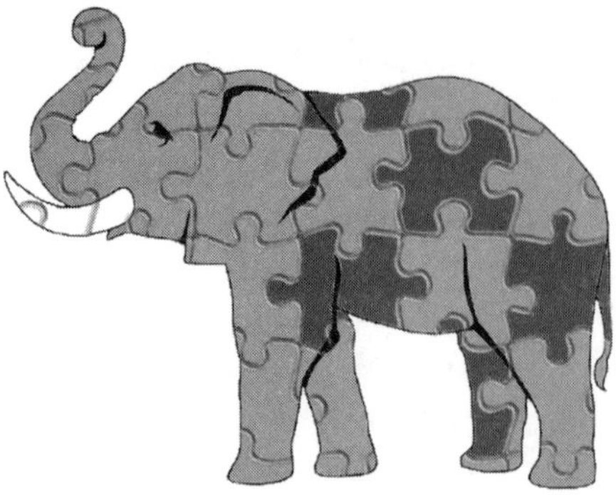

Chapter 5

Untreated Iron Overload Can Give You Heart Disease

Rhonda's undetected irregular heartbeat had progressed to heart failure that allowed a buildup of fluid throughout her body.

In another case, the patient's medical records described him as obese. Extreme fluid retention had been misinterpreted as obesity!

Iron reels chaotically from organ to organ, rusting out the interior as if it were a metal automobile. Vitamin C latches onto iron, binds with it and moves it around. Arthur Nienhuis, MD, reported in 1977 that vitamin C mobilizes iron into the heart muscle. (NEJM 1977 296:114).

Vitamin C taken with iron increases absorption of the iron. Patients who have discovered they are iron overloaded learn to drink orange juice in the midmorning instead of with breakfast.

Jerome L. Sullivan, MD, PhD, has written in the literature about his tantalizing hypothesis that excess iron can cause anybody to have a heart attack, not only those with the heart disease as a result of genetic hemochromatosis. We'll discuss Sullivan's theory later. One point he makes is that workers in England have reported that traces of iron greatly increase rhythm irregularities following heart attacks. At the same time an iron chelator, desferrioxamine, greatly decreases rhythm disturbances following coronary blockage. The chelator removes a bit of iron from the organ.

Sullivan makes the point that iron, "even at levels long regarded as normal, may have deleterious effects in the heart." (*Ironic Blood* Vol 6No 6). "Normal" levels should be lowered. Sullivan speaks of cholesterol. He says that "The notion that cholesterol is of central importance has become a rigid and institutionalized point of view." [J Clin Epidemiol Vol. 49, No.12. pp1345-1352, 1996]. In the same paper he counsels, "We have a duty to the public to understand and prevent ischemic heart disease even if it means rethinking old concepts." He points out that many hundreds of thousands die each year from heart disease. The cholesterol theory has taken such strong root in the scientific community that it reminds us of the now dreaded maleleuca tree that flourishes in Florida, but has been declared a harmful weed that causes widespread respiratory allergies and is now illegal to plant. New Maleleuca trees may not be planted, yet Florida neighborhoods are still filled with the pesky trees.

Charles F. Babbs, MD, PhD, at Purdue University conducted experiments in which animals achieved a doubling of long-term survival with the iron chelator given after six to ten minutes of total circulatory arrest. *(Annals of Emergency Medicine* Aug 1985).

"If iron overload imposes a risk [to heart injury] does normal iron sufficiency also impose a risk?" asks Joe M. McCord, PhD, in a March 1991 editorial in The American Heart Association's publication *Circulation.* He quotes from Sullivan's writings that since women's risk of heart disease increases after menopause, it may be menstrual blood loss, not estrogen levels that protect the heart from iron damage. He further quotes that "blood donation three times a year will lower the serum ferritin level of a man to that of a young woman." He concludes, "What may be bad news for the Geritol generation may be good news for the Red Cross."

We must look at iron with new eyes!

Opal in Midwest City, Oklahoma, was experiencing irregular heart rate and atrial fibrillation. Over the years she sought help from a variety of doctors and heart specialists. More than one said, "What's wrong with your liver?" She did not know. One day a physician took some blood to test for hepatitis. "No, Opal, it isn't hepatitis."

But no one followed up the swollen liver. Then she saw a new cardiologist. He squinted his eyes thoughtfully. "Did you spend all summer at the lake?" She had not. "Then why are you so brown in the winter?" She did not know. "Opal, I believe you are iron overloaded."

Opal gasped. She started remembering a gynecologist who had given her iron for anemia for twenty-eight years!

The diagnosis was made; the life was saved. Any malfunctioning heart is sending out a pulsating message: measure iron, measure iron.

A study from University of Utah by Corwin Q. Edwards, MD, and colleagues noted that there was less serious heart disease among patients in the study than is usually found. Edwards explained this by the fact that twenty-eight of the thirty-five patients had been diagnosed early because they were related to previously diagnosed patients. However, there were abnormalities that included atrial ectopic beats; atrial fibrillation; incomplete right bundle branch; low voltage and enlarged heart.

IOD receives constant reports of a variety of heart disease from the large patient network in its membership.

The view that blood donation may protect against heart disease was offered in Lab World, Aug 1981. Quoting Jerome Sullivan's paper in Lancet, June 13, 1981, the article said that heart failure incidence increases in iron storage diseases, that iron accumulates with age and that possibly normal serum ferritin levels have been set too high and should be "redefined."

Sullivan sees excess iron in the heart as a poison that causes arrhythmias and damage to the heart muscle. Supporting this view is the fact of the very low heart disease rates among poor people in third world countries, who are universally regarded as "iron deficient." This population eats high fiber diets that retard iron absorption and in addition the people are loaded with gastrointestinal parasites. But these people suffer the world's lowest rates of myocardial infarction.

A recent study shows that deficiencies of folic acid, B6 or B12 are associated with heart attacks. Supplying these deficiencies tends to reduce the levels of homocystine levels, which do the dirty work. Very interesting! As it happens these very same deficiencies result in iron-loading anemia. Don't just supply these deficiencies to help the heart. At the same time make sure to reduce the iron.

Despite decades of efforts in the U. S. to lower patients' cholesterol, deaths from heart disease continue to increase. Some of the very cholesterol reducing drugs actually increase mortality. Considering that the drugs kill rather than heal exposes a whole new subject about the corporate pharmaceutical community that is subject for another book.

Sullivan says plainly that the idea that high cholesterol is at the bottom of heart disease "has outlived its usefulness and should be discarded." Meanwhile it should be obvious that the role of iron has been virtually neglected.

Science has no use for "anecdotal evidence," but IOD nevertheless offers two decades of speaking hourly with physicians, scientists, and patients from all over the world, and we can see the connection between heart and iron as clearly as if it were written across the heavens. The daily aspirin regimen to protect the heart is generally accepted as valid. Why does aspirin work? It is also well known that when you take aspirin you are going to lose a little blood — (iron).

Why do laboratory rats that are fed a spare diet enjoy considerable more longevity than those permitted to eat at will? Again, less iron.

In these discussions Sullivan is not really speaking of iron overload. He is saying that *iron depletion* protects the heart. So this is everybody, not just hemochromatosis patients.

Sullivan's hypothesis received validation after a Finnish study in 1992. Jukka T Salonen MD PhD randomly selected 2,000 Finnish men. The subjects were examined and found to be free of any symptoms of coronary heart disease. Fifty-one of the men experienced acute myocardial infarction over three years. Those men with ferritin greater than 200 had a 2.2 fold risk factor, compared with men with lower serum ferritin. Most labs and most physicians consider 200 ferritin as perfectly normal.

The conclusion was that a high level of storage iron poses risk of heart damage. The study was the cover story of *US News and World Report* and received much media attention for a short while.

Studies and research are wonderful, but we now have enough information to save just about everyone's life, those with even a little too much iron. That's why, when a government bureaucracy wants to delay action "until we have more studies," we groan, "This will never happen in our lifetime."

After more than two decades of day and night work IOD was disheartened over and over by stories flooding in that made it clear that ignorance about iron was still the norm.

One day a knowledgeable physician sent a copy of a Case Record from *The New England Journal of Medicine* (Aug 18 1994). The sender was outraged at the calm acceptance of innumerable errors that were made in the case of a 25-year-old who had endured a heart transplant followed by a liver transplant.

The story says that the patient had been well until four months before this traumatic hospital admission. One more reason to know your iron level before body damage, before symptoms. A chart of laboratory values on the patient did show iron at 149 and Total Iron-Binding Capacity (TIBC) at 162. But the math was not done, there was no saturation listed. The math would have shown a 92 percent saturation. The report cited a long list of conditions that cause congestive heart failure. The list does include hemochromatosis. But the patient did not fit the picture of what doctors expected of a hemochromatosis patient. That word: hemochromatosis! It's killing people. Nobody really fits the picture. You are too young, too female, too fair-skinned, lacking diabetes. Does it really matter if the diagnosis is heeeeemohhhkrohhhmahtosis? **Iron** is what will kill you. Iron!

Because this young patient suffered heart and liver among other complications, physicians had scurried down this path and that path chasing this expensive possibility and that other.

Physicians who have treated hemochromatosis patients usually receive them close to end stage. They are older, sicker and not long for this world. That's hemochromatosis.

First the story said this particular patient had been well until four months before hospital admission. A little later in the story it was admitted that the young man had been evaluated three years earlier because of a variety of anemia and thrombocytopenia, in other words, anemia and low platelets. Doctors at that time examined his bone marrow, but found no reason for the abnormality. A bone marrow biopsy is not going to show iron levels. Right here, at this point, physicians should have measured iron, as a normal precautionary measure. But no one thought of it. He was told it might be Epstein-Barr.

Well, we hear that a lot, too. Epstein-Barr. It's as if let's make this more complicated than just something simple like too much iron. The truth is, iron was never thought of.

Finally, by the time the young man required major organ transplantation, he received a diagnosis. Because iron was the last cause thought of instead of the first, the patient had to endure the trauma of transplant of heart and liver, with all that entails, not to mention appalling medical cost.

Paul Cutler MD, a Niagara Falls physician spoke at IOD's 17th Annual Symposium in 1999. He told of four of his patients who had been put on a list for heart transplants. Cutler treated the patients with Desferal to reduce iron levels, and their hearts improved enough that the transplants were no longer needed. All four were taken off the heart transplant list.

Desferal is a drug that is infused over twelve hour periods while patients sleep. It is used for patients who are so anemic they require blood transfusions, and for that reason cannot give blood. Not as effective as bloodletting, Desferal has nevertheless saved many lives.

Most people who have iron caused heart disease are unaware of their iron overload.

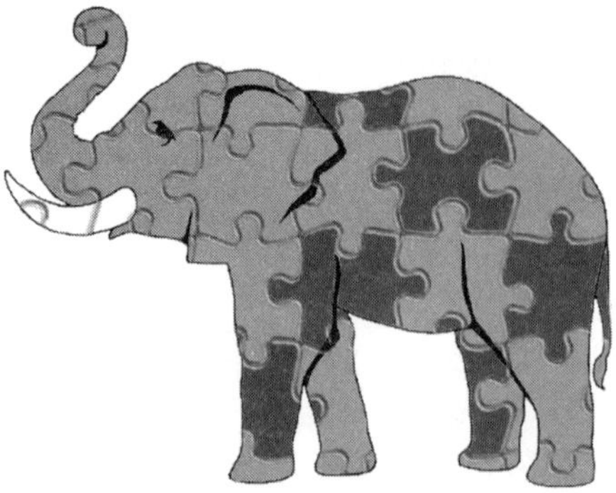

Chapter 6

Untreated Iron Overload Can Give You Cirrhosis

"Patient denies excessive use of alcohol," is frequently noted in medical records of liver patients. The individual who has a genetic defect in iron metabolism innocently eats his meals, not knowing he is poisoning himself by absorbing too much iron. The primary target organ for iron is usually the liver, which becomes overloaded and injured. Fibrous tissue may cause the liver to become inflamed and swollen. Or the opposite. The liver can shrink. It can become small and hard.

"Dear Sirs: I have hemochromatosis ... my mother's sister died of cirrhosis of the liver in her thirties. The doctor at the Cleveland Clinic thinks she probably had hemochromatosis..." writes Mrs. G. B. of Burbank,Ohio.

It is certain that many thousands of victims whose death certificates list cirrhosis or liver cancer as the cause of death were suffering undiagnosed hemochromatosis. The typical newly diagnosed patient recollects, "My mother (grandfather, uncle, brother) died of cirrhosis." The new patient logically speculates that the underlying cause of the earlier death was genetic iron overload.

The first patient I met was diagnosed in 1977 and never treated. He died two years later. The goal should be to detect all cases *before* cirrhosis develops. But without fail every cirrhotic patient must be carefully evaluated for iron levels. Cirrhosis is another flashing signal that says: check iron.

Older medical texts indexed hemochromatosis in the liver sections. It used to be considered a liver disease, and a few dreary paragraphs described the ailment as "fascinating but unfortunate." By the time it adds liver to its list of damage, hemochromatosis is indeed not the most fortunate of diseases. You may be wondering, since the liver is the target organ, why it would not cause the earliest symptoms. The liver is truly a heroic organ that detoxifies poisons and protects the entire body. It is capable of healing and regenerating itself and can withstand amazing punishment.

The liver is the largest of the body's organs, except for the skin. The liver has its work cut out for it. Everything that goes into the body, food, drink, air, must be processed by the liver. The liver stores a supply of nutrients needed for its business, and acts as a clearing house, cleaning the blood and sorting out wastes.

Hemochromatosis is not a liver disease. In later books you begin finding hemochromatosis in the hematology sections. But it is not a blood disease, either.

Hemochromatosis is a disease of faulty metabolism for iron.

Pete, a San Bernardino, California, businessman, went into the hospital for gall bladder surgery. Surgeons discovered that the gall bladder and surrounding ducts were "totally clogged with iron." They found the liver to be severely enlarged and full of iron. Pete received a lucky diagnosis at age fifty.

Walter G. Frey, III, MD, of Dartmouth, has written a recommendation that liver iron be quantified to guide therapy. Knowledge of the amount of iron to be unloaded is helpful in estimating the length of treatment. (NEJM 265:7-12 July 6, 1981). Frey expressed disappointment later that colleagues in medicine were slow to follow through on quantitative analysis. However such practice is now becoming more common.

A biopsy of the liver with appraisal of the amount of iron deposited still gives the most complete information of the individual's iron status. However most clinicians now feel that the biopsy is not essential to making the diagnosis.

Liver dysfunction leads to many problems including mental confusion. When the liver becomes overburdened or injured, it must work harder to metabolize certain substances such as alcohol, fats and protein.

"Early autopsy reports described patients with deafness, cerebellar and pyramidal signs with xanthochromic CSF, and hemochromatotic pigmentation of the meninges, cerebral cortex, olfactory bulbs, cerebellum, pons and the tectum of midbrain," wrote Naunihal Singh, MD, and colleagues [*Arch Neurol* - Vol 34, Feb 1977]. The authors gave a case report of a patient who had suffered unsteadiness of gait, slurred speech and uncoordination. The conclusion was that "the reversal of grossly abnormal EEG findings to normal in this patient, accompanying treatment, perhaps suggests that both the EEG changes and his cerebellar dysfunction resulted from hepatic encephalopathy." Encephalopathy is disease of the brain.

Despite earlier belief that iron could not cross the brain barrier, it is now known that iron can get into the brain, where it can in severe cases result in a condition called Hallervorden-Spatz. This disease affects young children, who gradually deteriorate and lose functions that are dependent on brain. These children lose mobility and vision and fail to develop and die before puberty.

In a variety of neurological diseases such as Parkinson's, multiple sclerosis, tardive dyskinesia, spastic paraplegia and Alzheimer's a bit of excess iron in the brain will cause more severity of disease and make the conditions more difficult to manage.

Iron in the brain was given prominent attention at an international symposium held in 1997 in France. Several presentations discussed brain lesions in multiple sclerosis in which there was found altered ferritin and transferrin distribution. Analysis had been made at autopsy of normal human brain tissue and of those diagnosed with MS. A "robust" presence of iron was found. It was suggested that iron plays a direct role in MS. IOD does know of numerous families with MS and iron overload.

Iron was found to be toxic to dopamine cells.

I have not heard of any success in removing the iron from the brain. But a way will have to be found. At the same meetings it was mentioned that it is necessary to determine whether iron chelation could help in the control of Parkinson's disease, for example.

At any rate, it can only help to give blood and lose iron from the body weekly so long as the hematocrit supports the treatment. A cutoff of 30 percent of the hematocrit is not too extreme. A little anemia will not kill you.

Tim, an Ohio man, young and healthy, died in an automobile accident. His generous family consented to have his organs donated to save life in other persons. Tim's family and his physician were unaware that Tim suffered hemochromatosis. The individual who received Tim's liver required a number of phlebotomies to rid the organ of the toxic iron. The liver would regenerate after the iron was removed. Tim's family was notified and his sister then received a diagnosis and treatment. The family remembered a grandfather who had died of cirrhosis and had been told he had too much iron. The fatal tragedy kept giving life after death. In more ways than one.

All members of an Alabama family were diagnosed as having hemochromatosis. Apparently both mother and father carried double genes for the condition. Last to receive a diagnosis was the mother, who was loading iron at a slower rate, but who nevertheless had developed cirrhosis. Her seven pregnancies may have protected her somewhat, slowing the rate of accumulation because of transfer of iron to the fetus.

Her eldest daughter did not receive an outright diagnosis, but was described as having elevated iron levels. She too had borne seven children.

In a Japanese study by Kichihei Miyasaki, MD, and colleagues, an autopsy of a sixty-eight-year old man revealed hemochromatosis. The patient had noticed neurologic symptoms six months before death. "Hemochromatosis is seldom associated with lesions of the brain," the authors said, "although there have been some reported cases in which this complication could not be considered accidental." The report noted there had been a slight elevation of blood ammonia recorded one month before death.

Some patients have reported to IOD a strong odor of ammonia in the urine.

J. Donald Ostrow, MD, spoke in May, 1982, to members of the American Liver Foundation meeting in Chicago. When protein is incompletely metabolized, he said, it allows a backing up of ammonia that can enter the brain and lead to headache, sometimes, severe, drowsiness, confusion, forgetfulness or difficulty with concentration.The patient can go into a coma or even die in extreme cases.

The encephalopathy was described as metabolic rather than organic by Donald Ritt, MD, speaking at the same meeting. He said the condition develops gradually with continual alterations in thought processes, progressing in extreme cases to coma. But hepatic coma leaves little permanent damage, he said, and the brain cell is structurally undamaged. Death from this event has been reported.

The doctors suggested that it would be helpful to decrease protein intake until the liver has improved.

If a liver biopsy is made, the specimen must be correctly examined and results have to be correctly interpreted before the patient can receive a correct diagnosis by biopsy.

Alyce of Prescott, Arizona, had been told for twelve years that her iron was elevated, even that her liver enzymes were elevated, but she did not hear the word hemochromatosis until nine years into the testing. At that time a doctor assured her she does not have the disease because the liver was not damaged enough.

Alyce requested a second opinion. The second doctor recommended immediate treatment.

Cirrhosis is not mandatory to confirm the diagnosis. Patients would rather *not* wait for the damage. Damage can be prevented.

Most people who suffer iron caused cirrhosis, whether or not they happen to suffer at the same time from alcoholism, are unaware of their iron overload.

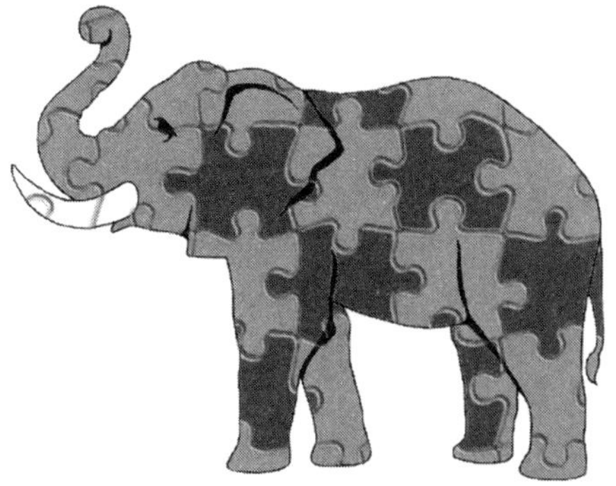

Chapter 7

Untreated Iron Overload Can Give You Diabetes

One day in her doctor's office in Mississippi Marta started feeling cold and colder. Nurses wrapped her in blankets, but she could not get warm. Finally a nurse had to bring a heater into the office and turn it full on Marta. The sudden temperature drop had happened before, but the doctor had not really believed Marta until this day. This day he hospitalized her. Hypothyroidism can be a complication of iron overload.

Looking back at those days, Marta rages that incompetent medical care — specifically medical ignorance about iron overload — has ruined her life. Her mother remembers her as a pretty little kid, a fair delicate-skinned redhead, lively but easily tired.

"If I had seen a Dr. Crosby at age fifteen," she says, "my life would have been different." Instead of being disabled, Marta is certain she would now be normal, with husband, children, career. William H. Crosby is a world-wide authority on hemochromatosis. Marta had met him at an IOD symposium.

At age twenty-nine Marta completed menopause and thus gave up her dreams of bearing children. Unsuccessful efforts to have a baby have scuttled many a marriage. Marta gave up on those efforts because of her many no-name illnesses.

Emotional scars deepened years later when a fiance jilted her just two weeks before their wedding. "Failing libido ... low energy ... it was too much for him," Marta says.

Health problems mounted. The act of eating became so strenuous that Marta would have to look for a place to lie down after meals. It was not that she neglected medical care. She allowed physicians to perform dilatation and curettage and two laparoscopies. She describes that procedure as "going in through the navel and looking around."

Marta started suffering a series of influenzes. "I never really got over one," she says, "they sort of overlapped." Doctors kept her on constant antibiotics, and for more than a year prescribed massive doses of Motrin for painful, crooked fingers. The medication did not help.

Profoundly exhausted and depressed, Marta visited her mother in Indiana for two weeks to recuperate. Friends were startled by her "greenish" color. Marta tried to help her color by sunbathing at poolside. Otherwise she slept for days and days. But Marta could not rest away the deep fatigue.

Back to Mississippi and back to doctors. "Well, your liver enzymes are elevated," said a doctor, "but if it were anything serious you'd be dead." When Marta asked for a second opinion, the doctor became defensive. "Why? You don't think I can take care of you?" Marta nevertheless sought help from an internist.

Finally a urine check revealed sugar. Diabetes was diagnosed. Iron overload was then detected at last. Marta's first migraine headache struck while she was in the hospital. Since then the headaches — "three day killers" — have become a weekly way of life.

Now Marta occupies herself with twice weekly phlebotomies to unload the iron and with managing her diabetes. She reflects on what has happened to her family. Her younger sister, Marybeth, working in television in New Jersey, then received a belated diagnosis as well. Marybeth's blood tests had also revealed elevated liver enzymes that were ignored. At age eleven Marybeth underwent treatment for hepatitis. The family's doctor was the same man who had treated their father, dead of a stroke, enlarged heart and enlarged liver at fifty-eight. His sickly brother had died at fifty-four; the father of the two brothers had died at fifty-five.

One thing that makes Marta grind her teeth is a notation she saw on medical records: "doubt hemochromatosis." This note was entered not once but twice over the years. Why was the suspicion not followed up? she cries.

Clinical manifestations of diabetes in a hemochromatosis patient are indistinguishable from those of any diabetes. Severity depends upon the amount of iron load and whether the diabetes is discovered early or late in the course of iron accumulation. You can expect improvement in about half of all patients when you unload the iron aggressively. Some patients are able to reduce or discontinue insulin injections. This outcome depends on the promptness of diagnosis. It depends on the vigor of therapy.

Diabetes is so often a feature of iron overload that an old-fashioned name for the disorder was "bronze diabetes." The term is not useful for two reasons. First not all patients do develop diabetes, and certainly not all patients are the bronze color that makes physicians secure in diagnosing. It is a mistake to rule out a diagnosis on the basis of either the lack of diabetes or a light skin.

Harold was a successful building contractor with an attractive wife and three sons. The family divided their time between Palm Beach and Bar Harbor, Maine. One day it happened. Harold received the unhappy diagnosis that he had diabetes. He was a man of means. He could afford the best in medical care, so Harold immediately checked in at the Joslin Clinic in Boston.

Blood sugar is difficult to regulate when the underlying cause of pancreas damage is excess iron, unless that iron is removed. Harold's doctors at the clinic did not ask, "is iron involved?"

It is preferable, of course, to find the iron before pancreas damage, but every diabetic should be carefully evaluated for iron. If you have diabetes and your iron levels are not measured, you are not receiving proper care. When physicians do not suspect iron overload, they do not look for it; when they do not look for iron overload, they do not find it.

The clinic gave Harold diet instructions and he went home to manage the diabetes. But the diabetes was unmanageable. Harold collapsed and ended in the hospital, where hemochromatosis was finally diagnosed.

Too late. Harold at that time had three months left of life.

Death certificates that list diabetes as the cause of death often omit the real underlying cause: hemochromatosis. No. The real cause is ignorance. You can successfully treat hemochromatosis when you detect it early.

Most people who suffer iron caused diabetes are unaware they are iron overloaded.

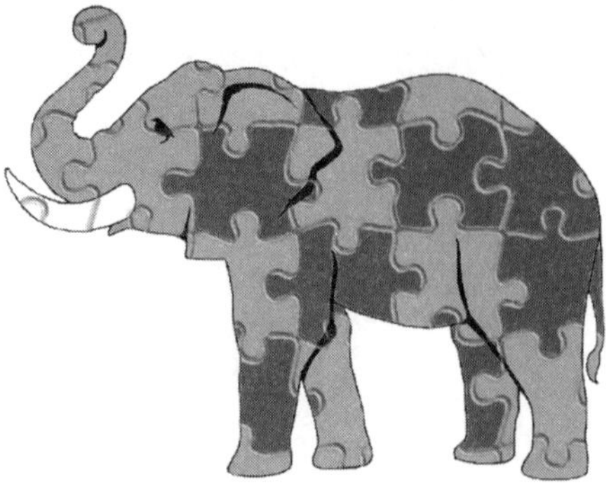

Chapter 8

Untreated Iron Overload Can Impair Your Immune System

One cruelly cold winter in Logansport, Indiana, where I worked as a radio copywriter, I caught a severe case of Asian flu. Every morning I woke up exhausted and was so weary I became too tired to eat. All that chewing and swallowing. Finally I dragged my ninety-five pounds to a doctor.

Her examination showed me to be "anemic" and "rundown." She prescribed iron.

Watching that scene now from this new perspective, I want to say, "No! Don't take it." The way you try to warn the victim in a gothic film not to open that door and walk into disaster.

Effects of flu lasted for more than a year. The cycles of flu, pneumonia, pleurisy, bronchitis and other evils that plagued me unceasingly were aggravated by the hidden excess iron in storage. Iron was accumulating secretly. Silently. Many patients have written to me of similar experience. If you have low resistance to colds and infection, if you are "run down," you may find the answer in lab reports of your iron readings. Everyone with depressed immunity should know his iron levels.

After the iron is unloaded, immune response greatly improves.

A fascinating discussion by Eugene D. Weinberg in BioScience Vol. 25, No. 5, describes the problems of a human body in attempting to withhold iron from invading bacteria. He refers to the action of raw egg white that helps stop dysentery growth, and remembers a passage in Shakespeare in King Lear, "I'll fetch some flax and whites of eggs to apply to his bleeding face." (Act III, Scene 7).

Weinberg goes on to note that egg white contains an anti-infective principle that must have been known to people in Shakespeare's time. He goes on to say that iron *neutralizes* the benefit of the egg white. In animal experiments endotoxin aided the animals' defense against bacteria. Later, Weinberg says, It was learned that endotoxin immediately lowers iron levels in circulation and also decreases absorption from food. Iron-stressed rats had one thousand times more bacteria in their kidneys than controls.

There is a "vigorous competition," Weinberg wrote, "between bacterial, fungal and protozoan pathogens....for the iron that is needed for (their) survival and growth." [*Biological Trace Element Research* 3,55-80 (1981)]. Weinberg pointed out that the body has a mechanism to "withhold iron from invading pathogens. This mechanism ...helps to protect, but the ability to withhold iron would be seriously impaired if the body is overloaded with iron."

Weinberg writes that people are much more susceptible to infections at times of high iron elevation. "Such persons," he says, "are also much more susceptible than normal members of their families or communities when exposed to identical kinds and quantities of pathogens."

Elsewhere, Weinberg said, historical evidence suggests that low body iron stores reduce mortality due to certain infectious diseases. Weinberg cited Ell SR. "Iron in Two Seventeenth Century Plague Epidemics" from *Journal of Interdisciplinary History* 15:445-57, 1985. *[Medical Hypotheses 21:441-443, 1986].*

The "boy in a plastic bubble" was kept alive for seventeen years. The boy had spent nine years at the National Institutes of Health in a sterile environment because of a breakdown in his immune system. He suffered aplastic anemia and required frequent blood transfusions to sustain life. The patient was successfully protected from infection, but he was not able to overcome the accumulation of iron that came with the transfusions. Keep in mind that many anemias are in themselves iron loading anemias. Aplastic anemia is one, and any anemia that is severe enough to require transfusions puts the patient on the road to a surplus of iron and to certain death *unless the iron is removed by chelation.* Such patients must make sure this life-saving support is given. The word chelation raises visions of alternative type medicine where EDTA is used presumably to remove plaque from veins to protect the heart. But chelation to remove iron is entirely different. IOD hears of EDTA being used for iron extraction, but EDTA is not effective for removing iron. Desferal is at this time the only FDA approved iron chelator.Not only is EDTA ineffective for removing iron, but it can be dangerous in iron overloaded patients, especially if vitamin C is added to the intravenous fluid, which is an unfortunate routine in EDTA chelation clinics. Paul Cutler MD, Niagara Falls, New York physician, has seen more than twelve iron overloaded patients made ill when given EDTA and vitamin C intravenously. They became ill from heart attacks, strokes or atrial fibrillation. In none of these cases did the chelating doctors order iron blood tests or suspect iron overload.

An imaginative description of how iron interferes with immunity was presented by William C. Douglass MD, in *Townsend Letter for Doctors.* "The chicken has an exquisite appreciation of the role that iron plays in infection," Douglass wrote. The yolk is rich in iron, but the egg white contains conalbumin, a powerful iron-binding protein, which is similar to transferrin, the iron-binding protein of blood. Bacteria have a tough time working through the barrier to the developing chick.

Douglass remarks that human mothers protect their breast-fed infants with lactoferrin, present in the milk. He says this is the reason breast-fed babies have a lower incidence of infection. Lactoferrin, unsaturated with iron, immobilizes bacteria by taking up the iron they need. This is explained in June Goodfield's *An Imagined World.*

Patients with rheumatoid arthritis are usually anemic, Douglass said, which may be another example of the body's withholding iron to defend against the arthritis. Bacteria and fungi eagerly accept iron, he said, and severe infection is the result.

"The normal response of the organism to an infection is to decrease the iron content of the blood," wrote Arturo R. Rolla MD [*Ironic Blood* Vol. 5 No. 3]. "Persons with hemochromatosis cannot do this well and the increased availability of iron makes them more susceptible to certain infections," he continued.

"This seems to be the reason why Vibrio vulnificus, a very virulent bacterium from the sea, has proven to be lethal to persons with an elevated level of iron in the blood, as in hemochromatosis, some chronic liver diseases and some chronic congenital forms of anemia. [No doubt the iron-loading anemias]. The Vibrio has been found in sea water, sediment, plankton and animals in eighty different sites of the Atlantic Seaboard, from Miami to Portland, Maine, as well as other parts of the world. Most of the time they were found in oysters and clams.

"One of the two known ways to acquire the disease is by eating uncooked seafood. Symptoms appear rapidly, on the average in fifteen hours. The Vibrio gains access to the bloodstream giving a picture of blood poisoning with a drop in blood pressure, shock and death.

"The other form is a skin infection from cleaning contaminated shell fish or from harvesting oysters and crabs. A small skin laceration rapidly becomes swollen, tender and red, with such a massive enlarging of the extremity that it may subsequently require amputation if appropriate treatment is not provided rapidly.

"Because this infection is associated with the sea, it tends to occur in coastal areas and during the warm months, May to October."

A Florida man did have a harrowing experience after exposure to raw oysters in the summer of 1983. This was before he had ever heard of iron overload, and in fact is what indirectly led to his diagnosis. He says he suffered all the symptoms described by Rolla. The attack was very nearly fatal on the second to third day. He recovered. His iron overload was detected by CAT scan. However, he says that he suffers lasting damage to his left leg. An occasional diagnosis is made by CAT scan or MRI.

"Even though the number of patients affected so far by the Vibrio vulnificus has remained very small," wrote Rolla, "most of the patients reported had an elevation in the blood iron level. If blood poisoning occurs, it has a mortality rate of forty percent." Occasionally alerts are issued along the coast, as epidemics flare up.

"There is an effective antibiotic treatment (penicillin and tetracycline) Rolla wrote, "but it has to be instituted promptly. The infection spreads rapidly so it becomes very important that the doctors start the antibiotic right away.

"Unfortunately this Vibrio is a new and very unusual germ, that is mostly unrecognized by doctors and laboratory personnel. The time it takes to identify it accurately may be too long.

"So it is recommended that persons with hemochromatosis avoid eating raw seafood and if they develop a picture of blood poisoning or an aggressive skin infection after being at the sea, their doctors should be alerted to this very unusual bacterium."

Since most affected people are unaware of their iron overload, it would be wise to treat raw seafood with caution. It would also be wise to know and monitor your iron levels.It is slowly being discovered that patients suffering a number of diseases would benefit by removing any excess iron. In addition to those well known, cirrhosis, diabetes, heart disease, cancer and on and on, iron is now implicated in AIDs, Alzheimers, SIDs, hepatitis, leukemia, multiple sclerosis, cystic fibrosis and Lou Gehrig's.

"The presence of iron makes (AIDs, Lou Gehrigís and cancer) progress much faster," says Joe McCord, after doing research at Webb-Waring Biomedical Institute in Denver. McCord predicts that "iron will be the cholesterol of the 1990s." He was over optimistic in the *awareness* of iron's danger, but I'll join him in predicting that iron will be the cholesterol of the new century.

Researchers at Hershey College of Medicine, Penn State, "have noticed that there is a lot of iron in the cells surrounding Alzheimers plaques." James R. Connor, PhD, Associate Professor of Neuroscience and Anatomy was planning studies to understand why cells in the brain accumulate iron and then to devise ways to block the iron.

At University of Toronto Donald MacLachlan MD divided 48 Alzheimers patients into two groups. Half received Desferal, the iron chelator. In that group their disease progressed only half as fast as the others. I'm wondering if the researchers realized how low the ferritin can be brought, for even better results.

A study at University of Calgary has isolated a bacterium protein that helps "steal iron from the body" and thereby deprive bacteria of the mineral in meningitis. Anthony Schryvers was working to develop a vaccine to combat the component common to all strains of the disease. Schryvers said that prevention is the only answer.

The HIV-infected body attempts to halt the onslaught by withholding iron from the pathogens. The iron burden is intensified by inhaling iron-laden tobacco smoke. The iron chelator, Desferal, has "retarded the progression of AIDs," says E. D. Weinberg, PhD, in a 1993 Conference on Iron and Microbial Iron Chelates in Brugge, Belgium.

In another paper (Am Soc Microbiology, Nov 1993) Weinberg said, although cells from Vibrio vulnificus "cannot multiply in normal human sera, they grow rapidly," when iron is readily available.

Weinberg notes that excessive iron in formulas given to infants under six months increases the risk of salmonellosis, botulism and SIDs. The lactoferrin in breast milk protects infants from excess iron. Up to 155 times as much iron is added to some formulas as is present naturally in breast milk. "Many studies on sudden infant death syndrome have cited non-breastfeeding as a primary risk factor." (J Trace Elements in Exp Medicine 7:000-000 1994)

Laura Sullivan MD, now practicing in Orlando, has discovered that when she lowers ferritin of hepatitis patients, their liver enzymes are reduced. A study reported in Int Med News and Cardio News (Aug 15 1994) shows that weekly phlebotomies of hepatitis C patients "not only brings down serum iron levels, it also reduces (liver enzymes) and hepatitis C virus levels." (Dr. Anna S. F. Lok and multiple investigators) observed that "high hepatic iron and serum ferritin ... predict poor response to interferron."

"High iron concentrations have been reported in the brains of multiple sclerosis victims," wrote Leslie S. Valberg, MD. (Can J Neuro Sci 1989). "High values were evident ... in patients whose condition was stable, as well as in those where it was deteriorating." White matter samples from MS brains show significantly higher concentrations of iron, calcium and zinc, as compared to controls. High iron values were found in eleven MS patients in a study of 31 females and 18 males, and appeared to be related to the severity of the disease.

The Lancet (Nov 1965) published a report of a study that showed "The absorption of iron salts was higher in the group of patients with cystic fibrosis". Researchers at University of Berne, Switzerland, found that "out of a total of 49 children who died of cystic fibrosis, 19 had considerable hemosiderosis of liver and spleen." Workers said, "There is no doubt that the pancreas plays a very important role in the regulation of iron metabolism, a more important one than is generally accepted." It concluded, "The absorption of iron salts by children with cystic fibrosis is without doubt far above the normal average."

Seven patients with varying psychiatric disorders tested with high iron and were treated with deferoxamine for seven to 22 weeks, which resulted in significant clinical improvement. (Paul Cutler MD Can J Psychiatry, Vol. 39, Feb 1994). "Iron plays a key role in many brain enzymes, specifically tyrosine hydroclase and phenylalanine hydoxylase," Cutler writes, "thus psychiatric disturbances caused by iron overload should not be unexpected.." Cutler says that "while internists argue over how much iron is 'too much', patients with hemochromatosis are being missed."

Cutler has also described benefits of phlebotomy to diabetics **who do not have hemochromatosis.**

Charles A. Thomas, Jr. PhD, Chairman of the Board at Pantox Laboratories in San Diego, said, "We think that high levels of body iron are a major contributor to degenerative disease."

Although the link is far from completely understood, there is clearly a link between high iron stores and infection and malignancy.

Your immune system is a vital element after receiving an organ transplant.

"Serum ferritin is a marker for a poor clinical course in certain forms of malignancy," writes Maria de Sousa to the editor of Lancet, Sept. 17, 1983. "A study of serum iron, transferrin saturation, and serum ferritin in transplanted (and AIDs) patients should help to clarify the transfusional iron load explanation for this intriguing form of immunosuppression that is beneficial to the survival of some, but not all, transplants."

As we know, doctors deliberately suppress the immune system

in transplant cases to prevent the individual's immunity from attacking the newly transplanted organ.

Baruch S. Blumberg is another person who has published studies regarding iron levels and the infection of the hepatitis B virus. He wrote that individuals with elevated iron levels may be more likely to develop detectable cancer of the liver than others. (*Proc. Natl. Acad. Sci. USA, Vol 78, No. 5 pp 3222-3224 May 1981*).

In another paper Blumberg wrote an editorial letter in reply to a suggestion by Maria de Sousa that iron panels should be studied in AIDs patients. Blumberg wrote "Ferritin itself has immunosuppressive effects and the increased ferritin concentration may also contribute to immunodeficiency."

Blumberg offered a proposal that has been found to be valuable. He wrote, "Can the replication of the virus be decreased by inhibiting the amount of iron (and/or ferritin) available to the host?"

And we can add that *removal* of iron has every prospect of benefiting the patient, at the same time, *doing no harm.*

In the *British Medical Journal* (1978;2:1113-5) M J Murray examined 137 iron-deficient Somali nomads. These people were treated with 900 mg ferrous sulfate or placebo for thirty days. They found that the iron-treated nomads had 36 infectious episodes while the placebo-treated had only six.

Despite numerous such studies published in many journals we know of almost no clinicians who consider lowering their patients' ferritin (with bloodletting) when they present with infections. It's also true that ferritin levels may be low already, the iron having been used up by the bacteria. The ferritin is usually not tested, but if it is tested and found to be elevated, hardly ever is any thought given to bringing down the level. Or if it is low, the physician is likely to prescribe more iron, which will only continue supplying the bacteria.

Remember antique medical texts showing barber chairs and leeches or the bleeding apparatus? Perhaps we should stop laughing at those medics, whose instincts were closer to what was needed.

When we say that too much iron will destroy your immunity, we are not trying to scare you to death. We say only that *untreated* iron overload can feed all kinds of bacteria, virus and parasites. Untreated. It's still true that a condition of having excess iron can be so benign that you would go out and choose this over many other deadly conditions. A surplus of iron is dangerous only when neglected. So be sure to find out if you have too much. If so, do not neglect it.

Most people with iron-caused impaired immunity are unaware of their iron overload.

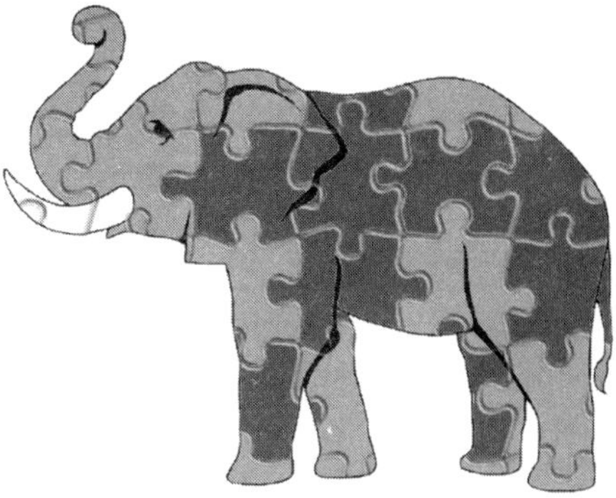

Chapter 9

Untreated Iron Overload Can Make You Tired, Tired, Tired

What a relief to the patient when he can put a name to the many random complex health problems that keep popping up. "I felt like the little kid who always yelled wolf," said Evelyn. The doctor who doesn't suspect iron will not order iron tests, or even worse, may believe that standard blood counts test iron. It's confusing to the patient's family. The patient complains of headaches today, yesterday it was stomach cramps, and before that his knees hurt. It's always something. "He doesn't look that sick," they say. They struggle to sympathize, but after all, the doctor found nothing wrong. Many a hemochromatosis patient receives a label of hypochondriac. He may be given tranquilizers; he may be sent to a psychiatrist. He begins to doubt his own perceptions. Psychiatrists need to be on the alert, as more than once, they have helped to lead the way to a correct diagnosis.

Looking back through your life, even at happiest times, your overwhelming memory is of tiredness. There's fatigue, there's tiredness, there's exhaustion. Ever try to tell a doctor that you're tired? Your listener can't hear you. You have pushed a button that brings an automatic if silent response. "Tired? Me too."

Fatigue is difficult if not impossible to measure. You spend years trying to deny it. Fatigue brings with it a feeling of guilt. When is it fatigue and when is it laziness? If everyone's tired, but other people can manage to keep going, why can't you? How do they do it?

"Don't you ever smile?" you keep hearing. Fatigue makes your face numb. You look at the clock and count the hours before you can lay down your head. Your eyes become marbles. Somewhere behind your eyes your mind starts closing down, even as you work at your desk. Forcing labor becomes a sort of preview of hell when you're tired, tired, tired.

Corwin Q. Edwards, MD, with colleagues wrote a paper on Thyroid Disease in Hemochromatosis, Increased Incidence in Homozygous Men, in which he reported a study of forty-nine patients. (Homozygous means the men possessed two genes for a recessive disease). "Our study has shown an increased frequency of thyroid disease in men who are homozygous for hemochromatosis," Edwards wrote.

"Physicians caring for patients with hemochromatosis should be aware of the high associated incidence of thyroid dysfunction." [Arch Intern Med - Vol 143, oct 1983].

In another report an Argentinian physician wrote, "an autopsy study of a large series of patients with hemochromatosis showed uniform infiltration of the parathyroid glands with iron."

Carlos A. Mautalen said, "Decreased parathyroid function is probably underdiagnosed in patients with iron storage disease." *[The American Journal of the Medical Sciences, Nov-Dec 1978 Vol 276 No 3].*

In recent years a whole new disease has surfaced, called Chronic Fatigue. I predict that sometime during the new Century a better understanding of where iron fits in human health will make a difference, such a difference that every symptom of iron surplus will not become highlighted as a separate disease.

Hemochromatosis is highly individual. Some patients do escape the fatigue and other complications until end stage. It is important to emphasize this in case a reader is too quick to breathe a sigh of relief and to murmur, "That lets me off the hook."

Let's hope it's true that you are in the clear. But someone you know, a friend, a relative, *someone*, is in desperate need of a timely warning. You may be in a position to save a life.

Many people whose fatigue is iron caused are likely to attribute their tiredness to anemia. They may indeed be anemic, but it is not iron deficiency. Anemia needs to be differentiated. Iron deficiency anemia is not all one word.

Pat, a San Diego woman, began treatment to unload excess iron. Her new sense of well-being and infusion of energy were a revelation. "I didn't know you were supposed to feel this good," she said. You cannot appreciate how tired you were until you begin to feel better and can compare now with then.

Most people with iron caused fatigue are unaware of their iron overload.

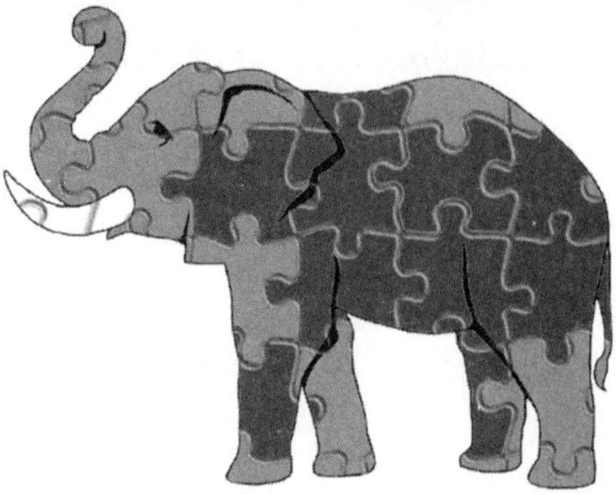

Chapter 10

Detected Early, Treated Properly, Iron Overload Leaves You Without Complications

Some patients are extremely lucky. Their iron overload is detected and removed, and they suffer none of what we have been discussing. Don't tell Katherine, though, that she's lucky. "What's lucky about being told you have a dreadful disease?" she wails. She hears "you're lucky" a lot and she hates it.

Katherine isn't crazy about the treatment either. Weekly bloodlettings are not a great deal of fun. But the point is she does it. And she keeps at it despite the fact that she feels well, has no symptoms.

Katherine's case is somewhat unusual in that her excess iron was detected early without advance diagnosis of a relative. She had suffered a violent reaction after dining on shellfish — and during examination her iron overload had surfaced. Katherine was purely lucky. But don't tell her I said so.

Katherine is unusual in another way. She could never be convinced that, feeling well, she had a terrible disease no one ever heard of. Subconsciously she wanted a doctor to say to her, "Nonsense, you don't have this disease." She kept visiting doctors until she found one who said just that. Surprisingly, the doctor's words failed to reassure. Logic took over. If you ever want proof that your body is storing too much iron, try bleeding out a pint a week. It's an impossibility unless you have excess storage iron available to make replacement blood. The ability to withstand weekly blood loss while not becoming severely anemic, proves iron overload.

"Without therapy, idiopathic hemochromatosis is a fatal disease," wrote Thomas H. Bothwell, MD, from Johannesburg, South Africa. "Death usually results from cardiac failure in younger patients and from liver disease or its complications in older ones. Some subjects succumb to an acute abdominal crisis followed by shock." [*Medicine,* Fifteenth Edition, 1979, Beeson-McDermott, pub. Wyngaarden].

It was excess iron that triggered the injury that ended the lives of those who carried the genetically predetermined condition.

This gloomy picture is beginning to brighten. Corwin Q. Edwards, MD, and his colleagues wrote that because of family studies patients are being found earlier. "In the past," he wrote, "most homozygotes have had heavy tissue iron loading at the time of diagnosis and were ill as a result. With increasing use of pedigree studies and the recognition of the value of simple laboratory screening tests, homozygous individuals are now being detected before any clinical manifestations develop. Thus it is no longer valid to expect individuals homozygous for the haemochromatosis gene to present with the classic triad of skin pigmentation, hepatomegaly and diabetes mellitus (bronze diabetes with cirrhosis)." [*Clinics in Haematology* Vol. 11, No. 2 June 1982]. Actually, it never was valid.

It's possible that you'll ring bells and buzzers at security check points. A reader of our newsletter was invited to the White House to accept an award. When he entered his body set off the alarm buzzers. Security people checked him out thoroughly with a "fine tooth comb," but they finally had to say, "You just have a magnetic personality." This happened to the man before his diagnosis. We'd like all security people to recognize that iron in the liver can cause a clatter, and we'd like the guards to advise those individuals to go have their iron tested.

Shirley in Oklahoma remembers that her husband rang buzzers at the Denver airport in 1983. It was not until 1991 that the man knew that he was dying of "this strange unknown disease."

Titanium joint replacements can set off the same alarms. One of the speakers at IOD's Tenth annual symposium almost didn't make it to the meeting because of delays at airport security. Titanium hips.

In 1991 a man died of excess iron at age 66. His grieving son copied IOD's fact sheet and distributed it at the funeral. A new diagnosis resulted.

For a rotten, deadly, hellish disease that kills you after exhausting your life savings, hemochromatosis is really a rather nice disease. One you'd go out and choose. It's nice because you'll know exactly what to do. Treatment is entirely effective. It requires no dangerous medicines. It's well-known that all medicines inflict side effects. The treatment is inexpensive — and should be free at the blood bank. And if you are motivated to unload the iron as fast as possible and keep it unloaded, you're likely to be healthier than average. Most people carry around a little too much iron.

However, be sure not to select this disorder and then neglect it.Don't be as unlucky as a man in Portsmouth New Hampshire, who died three days after diagnosis. For three months the patient had been under "close treatment" for cancer. No thought given to why the cancer. No testing for iron — until end stage. The physician said, "This is so rare we had a difficult time finding the source of the cancer."

We are asking doctors not to wait for body damage. We are saying to them, "You have been misinformed. Iron overload is not rare. It is common. You are missing the diagnosis and letting your patients die in front of your eyes." We are saying, "Please test the iron of every patient and don't be satisfied if the iron is only a little elevated. Protect your patients from iron's toxicity."

And we say to patients, "Don't put your life in the hands of a physician. Be sure you know your iron level, and be sure it is low or get it low. Take charge of your own health."

You are not looking to be diagnosed with a *disease.* You are testing *iron.* Disease or not, a small surplus of iron can cause a variety of damage throughout the body. Your goal is to prevent even a little iron rust irritating any of your body parts.

Katherine's kind of good luck is devoutly wished for the one and a quarter million Americans living on a kind of death row, unknowingly carrying within themselves ticking time bombs, not to mention 43 million single gene carriers and not to mention anybody else with iron overload for whatever reason.

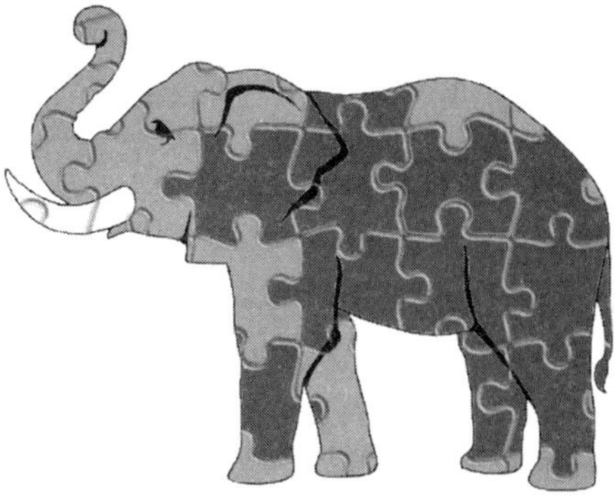

PART 2

"I've never heard of it, so how common can it be?"

Chapter 11

Hemochromatosis Is One Of The Most Common Genetic Diseases

Patients describe their frustrating experiences while searching for answers to medical problems. Their health was falling apart and they turned to physicians for help. When patients asked their doctors to check iron levels, "it's rare, you don't have to worry," has been a typical reply.

Those physicians were twice wrong. The individual with a rare disorder requires a correct diagnosis urgently when the rare disorder is treatable and the alternative to early detection is death.

The second is a scandalous wrong that has cost innumerable lives. Iron overload is not a rare condition; it's common.

Virgil Fairbanks, MD, Mayo Clinic internist, charged in a crisply critical paper that the incidence of hemochromatosis amounts to an epidemic. [Mayo Proceedings 61:296-298, 1986]. What incidence justifies the word "epidemic?" Webster's Third New International Dictionary Unabridged defines epidemic as: affecting many persons in a community. The many persons who are affected don't have to *know* they harbor a disease for it to be an epidemic. Andrew Dean, MD, of the Center for Disease Control gave a precise definition from the Dictionary of Epidemiology, Oxford Press, 1983. " ...occurrence in a community or region of cases of an illness ... clearly in excess of normal expectancy."

One in two hundred people with double genes for the abnormality and one in eight carrying the single genes qualify the disorder as an epidemic. Someone you know is affected — knowingly or unknowingly.

Are you asking whether everyone with the double genes will come down with the disease? Perhaps not. Think of the great variation in rates of iron absorption. Rhonda had not medicated with iron, yet she absorbed enough iron from ordinary food to kill her at twenty-three. At the same time others who were heavily iron medicated are still alive in the fifties, sixties and beyond.

Everyone absorbs iron at a different rate. Does this possibly include people with "normal" iron absorption? Those with normal iron metabolism have nevertheless been found to resist infection better when their iron stores are low.

Getting back to "will all double gene carriers develop full-blown disease?" The answer is no. Not if early detection and adequate treatment prevent injury. The excess iron must be recognized at whatever decade of life it appears and must be promptly removed, without waiting for "disease." The disease in that sense is preventable.

"One most serious misconception," writes William H. Crosby, MD, "is that a diagnosis of hemochromatosis can be made only when the disease is fully developed." [Arch Intern Med, Vol 146, June 1986].

Hemochromatosis is by far the most common of the iron overload diseases. Others include:

thalassemia
porphyria
sideroblastic anemias
pyridoxine-responsive anemia
hereditary spherocytosis
glucose-6-phosphate-dehydrogenase-deficiency
alpha 1 anti-trypsin syndrome

dietary iron overload
iron medication-induced overload
maintenance hemodialysis
postportacaval shunt surgery
Hallervorden-spatz (iron in the brain)

Look at the anemias in that list and you'll see why it's dangerous to medicate with iron just because you are anemic. No woman should allow her doctor to do this to her. If she is unwilling to insist that her physician investigate to differentiate her anemia, she may be better off living with the anemia. It is true that some anemias are life-threatening, and some of those listed do require treatment, but not with iron. They require iron removal! Adding more iron will hasten the patient's death. The only anemia that improves after iron medication is iron deficiency anemia. Even in that instance it is essential to investigate for the blood loss that is the probable cause of the low iron level.

Hemochromatosis is the traditional term for the most common of the iron overload diseases. The name was given by von Recklinghausen almost one hundred years ago.

It is an inexact, nondescriptive term, indeed a bad word,because it does harm. To receive a diagnosis of "hemochromatosis" according to recent medical definitions, you must have liver cirrhosis, heart enlargement and diabetes, or a "classic triad" described in some texts as liver cirrhosis, heart disease and skin pigmentation. The patient is not well served if he must wait for body destruction before beginning treatment. This kind of damage can be prevented.

We must learn to think of excess iron as a toxic substance to be removed. We can avoid body damage by looking at iron with new eyes. Think of iron this way: if the body is storing excess iron, we must unload the excess and avoid injury. We can then say we have prevented hemochromatosis. Or say that you managed early hemochromatosis.

If we can agree that hemochromatosis, early or late stage, exists, regardless of the amount of injury, we free ourselves from the necessity of seeing ruined body parts before making the diagnosis. We can then use the term "hemochromatosis" safely.

"The hemochromatosis gene is thirty times more prevalent than that for Duchenne muscular dystrophy," said Corwin Q. Edwards, MD, in a paper in 1987 at American Gastroenterological Association symposium. More than a million people have been diagnosed in the United States with disorders from a group of neuromuscular diseases.

The National Institute of Neurological and Communicative Disorders and Stroke published the following incidences of some well-publicized diseases in the U. S.

Cerebral palsy, 750,000 diagnosed cases, 9,000 cases per year

Multiple sclerosis, 137,000 diagnosed cases, 8,000 cases per year

Cystic fibrosis, 20,000 to 30,000 — 1 of every 1,600 newborns

The United States government has spent $45.8 million in research money for cerebral palsy and $27.5 million for multiple sclerosis.

The National Institute of Diabetes and Digestive and Kidney Diseases (NIDDKD) estimates that one in twenty Americans is a carrier of the single gene for cystic fibrosis, twelve million total. the National Heart, Lung, and Blood Institute says, "Because of the high incidence of CF, there is an urgent need for safe and reliable tests to rule out carrier status for the CF gene and for early and accurate determination during pregnancy of whether the fetus at risk will be born with the disease." [NIDDK 1987].

The reason hemochromatosis is not receiving similar attention with its estimated *forty-two million* single gene carriers is that the enormous cost of iron overload in lives and fortunes has until recently gone unrecognized. Awareness is missing. The condition is buried in icebergs underneath our very feet. The irony is that hemochromatosis is *treatable.* The terrible cost is avoidable.

The hemochromatosis gene is probably the most common abnormal disease-causing gene known. This should not be surprising since the diseases that result are the most common suffered by humans: arthritis, cancer, heart disease, diabetes, cirrhosis. In a large number of people suffering from these miseries, excess iron is the underlying cause. The growing awareness of the proper place of iron in human health — and the awareness has started — will bring a benefit similar to other signal advances in medicine.

Vincent Felitti MD, director of Kaiser Permanente's Preventive Health Care program at the HMO finds the present situation disturbing. "Once one begins looking, it is both startling and embarrassing to see how common hemochromatosis is," he says.

Diseases from recessive genes have traditionally been presumed to be rare, since the patient has to inherit a double set of genes, one from the mother and one from the father. A coincidence must exist, that two single gene carriers marry and produce children with both genes. In this setting, successive generations are not affected unless they marry gene carriers. Neither parent will be affected, as they are carriers only, although newer information is being unearthed that anyone with the single gene may suffer a variety of body injury from increased iron levels.

Paul Cutler said at IOD's 17th Annual symposium, "The concept that heterozygotes don't get ill is wrong." He said, "Doctors love to sweep iron under the carpet."

Walter G. Frey, III, MD, Professor of Medicine at Dartmouth Medical School, treated four generations in a single family. "I had decided that hemochromatosis had to be dominant rather than recessive inheritance," he told an audience at a medical symposium sponsored by IOD in 1984, "because you just wouldn't find the disease in four successive generations." This would be the case for all other recessively inherited diseases.

However, Frey explained, the disease certainly is recessively inherited. The explanation for the four successive generations Frey treated is that the gene is so widely prevalent, so common, that each generation married into a gene pool of carriers.

In Florida two half brothers were diagnosed. The mother, with the silent single gene, married twice, each time a husband who also carried the single gene. With any other recessive disease, such a happening would be a rarity, an oddity.

All nine members of an Alabama family have been identified with hemochromatosis. Both parents carry both genes and all seven children are affected.

IOD recently learned of an Irish couple, husband and wife, who are both diagnosed. Someone on the internet made a claim that the prevalence in Ireland is much greater than anywhere else. A report was published in 1998 in *Blood Cells, Molecules and Diseases.* Authors of the study included Eleanor Ryan, Conor O'Keane and John Crowe. Dr Crowe works at Mater Hospital in Dublin. The study shows that one in 100 Irish carry both copies of the HFE gene. An additional twenty percent of Irish carry the single gene, one in five people.

A study of sixty spouses of patients revealed an even higher rate of thirty-three percent (one in three). In the U. S. 170,000 people have immigrated directly from the Irish Isles. In that population the above incidence figures would apply. Among Americans are thirty-nine million who claim Irish ancestry. The incidence of the HFE double gene in that group is expected to be somewhere between the general population of one in 200 and one in 100. And the single gene incidence is somewhere between one in five and one in 7.5.

Iron overload can no longer be called a "disease of Caucasians." Victor Gordeuk MD, professor of medicine at George Washington University in Washington, has made a study of Africans and African-Americans. He finds their gene frequency appears to be one in 100, twice the incidence of others. And much less often diagnosed.

Family studies in several countries have led to estimates of a gene frequency of three per thousand persons (homozygotes, having both genes) in France. Studies in Australia yielded an estimate of eight per thousand. Previous estimates were much less. However, those estimates were based on the numbers of recognized cases seen in hospitals.

University of Utah studies projected estimates of five per thousand, and the same was found in Sweden. Estimates of heterozygote (single gene carrier) incidence in French studies stood at ten percent of the population, while in Australia it was sixteen percent. The location of the study is not believed to be a factor, since it is becoming clear that iron overload can affect all races and nationalities and both sexes and can be severe enough to kill at any age, including newborn, even not yet born.

Marcel Simon, MD, spoke at a 1987 Conference of Hemochromatosis sponsored by the New York Academy of

Sciences. Simon insisted several times that "the French are different." *C'est possible.* The gene itself was not identified, at that time, only gene markers. Much work had to be done in the understanding of the inheritance and its variabilities.

A chart of genetic prevalence was presented by Corwin Q. Edwards, MD, at annual meetings of American College of Physicians in 1985 and 1986.

	Heterozygosity percent	Homozygosity per 1000
Beaumont et al (France)	10	3
Dadone et al (Utah)	13	5
Bassett et al (Australia)	16	8
Olsson et al (Sweden)	13	5

"...almost always hemochromatosis has been surprise autopsy diagnosis," said Conrad Lundblad, MD, in Minnesota Medicine (58-3, 1975).

Although less common, the other iron overload diseases also take their toll. The thalassemias are a type of iron loading anemia, the most serious being thalassemia major or Cooley's anemia. These diseases are most prevalent among people of Mediterranean origin. They also occur in Asian people. In the severest form, children barely survive into their twenties. Patients must receive blood transfusions, which deposit large amounts of iron in their tissue, which is especially damaging to the young hearts.

The genetic defect causes abnormalities in the red blood cell (RBC). Its shape, size and color may be abnormal. The RBC is fragile and breaks down before its usual one hundred twenty days. When the red cells die they release iron into the blood-making mechanism. The shorter the life span of the cell, the bigger the iron storage deposition becomes. The iron stores that accumulate in these patients create a difficult problem.

Desferal, a chelator that binds with the iron and causes a small amount to be excreted, is usually administered to extend the lives of these patients.

Researchers in England found that iron overloaded patients were usually vitamin C deficient. Using the vitamin in combination with an iron chelator has made possible much more removal of iron in urinary excretion.

However, Arthur W. Nienhuis, MD, has cautioned from the National Institutes of Health that care must be taken, as vitamin C can mobilize iron into the heart muscle.

Iron overload is found in patients with porphyria cutanea tarda (PCT). The skin becomes affected with bulbous lesions, which are made much worse by sunlight. In a discussion by Mark L. Bassett, MB, June Halliday, MD,PhD, and Lawrie W. Powell, MD, PhD, phlebotomy therapy was recommended. "Phlebotomy therapy often results in a rapid clinical and biochemical remission," said the authors, "although the mechanism is poorly understood. Phlebotomy may even be useful in patients with increased hepatic iron stores." Suggested was the weekly removal of five hundred milliliters of blood until the urinary uroporphyrin excretion approaches normal or the hemoglobin falls below eleven. The patient should also avoid sunlight and alcohol.

Factors that activate this disease include excess iron intake, alcohol or estrogen. The patient may suffer skin outbreaks of scabby crusts, darkening or lightening color, areas of excess hair and possibly disfiguring of ears, nose or fingers.

In the porphyrias there is an overproduction of porphyrin precursors and storage of excess uroporphyrin in the cells of the liver. Porphyrins are chemical precursors of a portion of hemoglobin. Malnutrition or inadequate intake of carbohydrates may aggravate the condition. There is a connection between porphyrin metabolism and zinc, and porphyrins are excreted in combination with zinc. The metabolic defect leading to some of the porphyrias has not been defined.

As in hemochromatosis, practitioners have been too quick to point to alcohol as a cause of symptoms in patients.

A danger faced by persons with even mild anemia is that doctors may medicate them with iron. In sideroblastic anemia (SA), iron loading is already part of the picture. Sideroblastic means: a young red cell still containing a nucleus. The patient will benefit from bleeding, if the anemia is mild, or from iron chelation therapy if transfusions are necessary. Administering iron will only worsen the patient's outcome.

SA is a disorder that usually occurs after middle age. However, it can affect young people. The genetic abnormality is often associated with hemochromatosis, and both disorders are found in various members of the same family. More males than females are affected, and males usually experience more severe disease.

Diagnosis is made on the basis of abnormal or ringed sideroblasts from bone marrow specimen. The patient is often without symptoms until the iron burden becomes great. As in hemochromatosis, iron absorption is excessive. The physician must not overlook the iron status of the individual with SA. The degree of anemia does not correlate with the severity of the iron load.

Sylvia S. Bottomley,MD, Professor of Medicine at University of Oklahoma, specializes in these anemias. She advises, "In about one-third of patients with the hereditary type, and very rarely in cases with the acquired type, the anemias can be considerably improved if not nearly corrected by vitamin B6 (pyridoxine) supplementation." She urges, "Any degree of iron overload must be established and treated. In persons with mild anemia the iron excess is easily removed with appropriately scheduled and supervised phlebotomies despite the anemia. Those needing regular transfusions must be treated with desferrioxamine, an effective and safe iron chelating agent, although requiring compliance and commitment by the patient and physician respectively."

Patients seek help from IOD for polycythemia, and IOD responds, although polycythemia vera and the acquired polycythemias are not iron loading diseases. The treatment is similar, because the excessive supply of red blood cells is relieved by bleeding. Hemoglobin levels may exceed 18 gm in males and 16 in women, and the hematocrit is usually above 54 percent in men and 49 percent in women.

Patients can prevent thrombosis and hemorrhage and extend life with proper treatment. Polycythemia vera sometimes progresses to leukemia. Other forms of polycythemia do not. An individual can acquire one kind of polycythemia from heavy smoking, due to excess carbon monoxide, or from emphysema, often caused by smoking.

Even animals are not exempt from iron overload. L. N. Johnston, a Tulsa Oklahoma veterinarian, has observed the effects of excess iron in older horses. "No doubt we see iron overload in animals and miss it," Johnston said, "just as doctors do in human medicine." He added, "The horsemen sure like to use a lot of iron in their horse food and I think I can see the ill effect in the older animals."

Johnston calls iron overload "the sly fox of medicine." He criticizes giving iron to dogs suffering hook worm anemia. "Take care of the parasites," he says, "and everything will take care of itself."

At a recent IOD symposium Johnston mentioned that birds seem to absorb iron more readily than mammals. He told of 23 Oklahoma ostriches that were fed food that was too iron-rich, and on post-mortem were found to have iron toxicity. He advised pet owners to check iron content of bird food "or even make your own," he said.

Cattle siderosis was found in a section of New Zealand where water has exceptionally high iron content. Cattle were staggering and dying in the fields from iron overload. [Clinics in Haematology 2:383 RW Charlton et al 1973]. A bull with hemochromatosis has been reported in University of California, Davis, School of Veterinary Medicine.

A letter to IOD from the owner of a macaw told of her bird's diagnosis of hemochromatosis. Solomon had stopped eating, singing and talking. The family was greatly concerned, until treatment with phlebotomies restored the bird's appetite and good humor.

A professor of pathology at University of California, San Diego, Dr Kurt Benirschke, is finding hemochromatosis among animals at the famous San Diego zoo. Lemurs were dying and monkeys were becoming affected. The doctor said it was all caused by the unnatural diet too high in iron and vitamin C.

Despite evidence of a high prevalence of hemochromatosis,

doctors have been slow to recognize the magnitude of the problem. A diagnosis is still a rarity. Fairbanks terms the high incidence "an epidemic" and writes, "yet most hemochromatosis is still diagnosed more often at autopsy than during life."

The estimated prevalence of hemochromatosis gene carriers was prepared by IOD, based on the population of the United States as reported in 1990. See the Table after the photographs.

Well, the long-awaited gene discovery was finally made in 1996. Great Excitement! Unfortunately problems emerged immediately. People who were obviously overloaded had only the single gene, or had none of the mutations identified. Their physicians stopped treating them! IOD had to counsel against even testing DNA. I had to keep saying that the gene isn't what's killing you. It's the iron! In August 1998 The Centers for Disease Control's Sharon McDonnell, MD., MPH, announced the CDC's decision not to recommend universal genetic testing. The study was published in the October 1998 *Annals of Internal Medicine.* Barbara Chapman wrote a lengthy article in CAP TODAY, journal of College of American Pathologists. Dr. McDonnell said, "We're working under the assumption that if your transferrin saturation is elevated, you're probably at greater risk of iron overload than if you just have a positive gene test."

Vincent J. Felitti, MD, agrees. In his screening program at Kaiser Permanent he is so far finding one in 250 people needing excess iron removed. He said, "in many parts of the country these individuals enter into a really chaotic situation." To gain patient's compliance and motivation, he presents each person diagnosed with a copy of *The Iron Elephant.* He also said that liver biopsy is not necessary to make the diagnosis. The blood tests are simple, reliable, and inexpensive, and the treatment confirms the diagnosis.

David Witte MD, PhD, director of Laboratory Control Limited in Ottumwa Iowa, in the same article spoke of the extremely high medical cost of the wide-spread failure in diagnosis. "If 10,000 asymptomatic individuals were screened and those with the disease treated were compared with 10,000 persons not identified until symptoms developed, the health care expense would be far less for those treated before symptoms were present." He said, "A screening test can be done for almost no money. The reagent for the first test costs two cents. He said, "One approach is to measure unsaturated iron binding capacity - a simple and easily automated way to identify those most likely to have elevated transferrin saturation."

Concerning genetic testing, Jerome Sullivan, MD, PhD, said, "Results of the gene test will confirm but will not exclude the diagnosis."

"So you've made a discovery?" is a small folder printed by Eugene D. Weinberg, PhD. He "respectfully submits to the scientific community the following checklist." Check one:

___It cannot be true because we were not taught it in school.
___It cannot be true because otherwise it already would have been discovered.
___It already has been known for quite some time.
___It is so trivial that it is not worthy of notice.
___It cannot be true because it is too simple.
___It cannot be true because the discoverer is an idiot.
___It cannot be true because it contravenes my ideas.

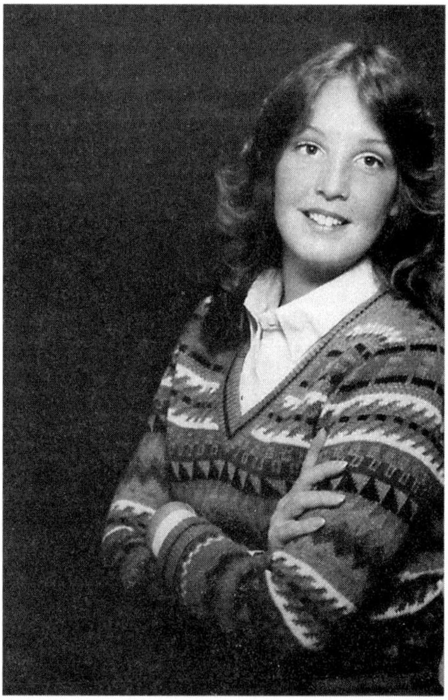

Rhonda Forman is shown at 17, right. Below are William H Crosby MD, an early leader in creating awareness of hemochromatosis in the medical community, with Rhonda's mother, Dolores Forman.

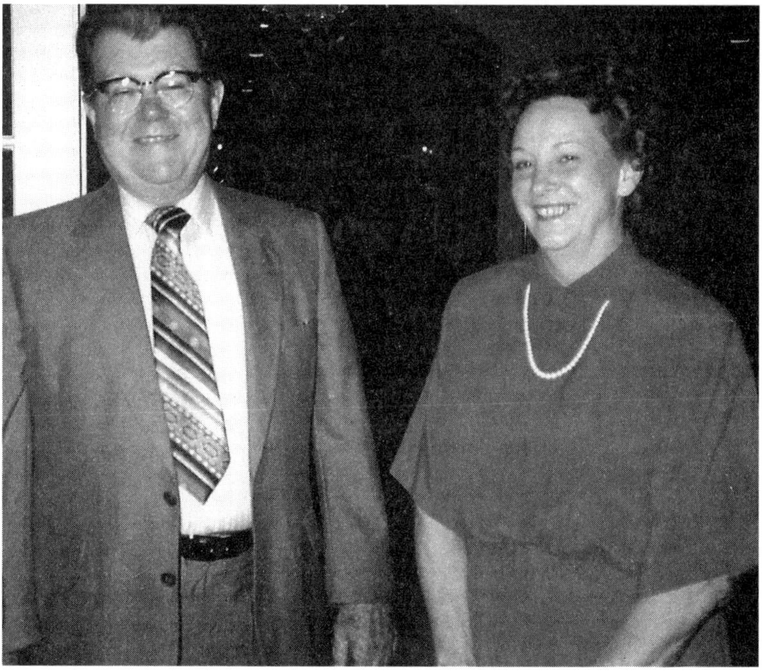

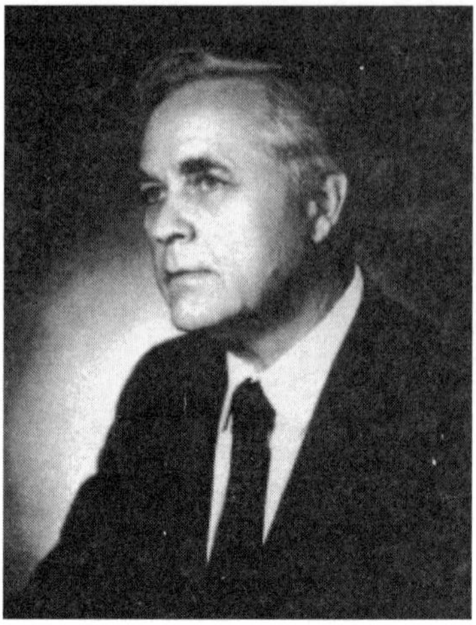

Virgil F Fairbanks MD, expert on iron overload at Mayo Clinic says, "Every case (of hemochromatosis) should have been diagnosed and treated early."

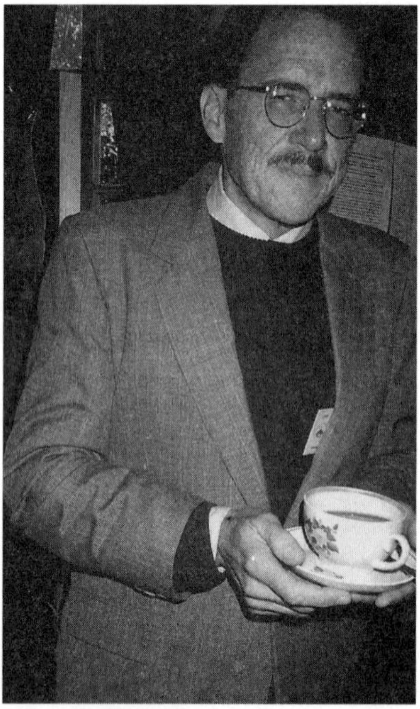

Victor Gordeuk MD speaking at the International Symposium on Erythron and Iron in Ryazan Russia in 1995. He pursues studies on the surprising incidence of iron overload in Africans and African-Americans.

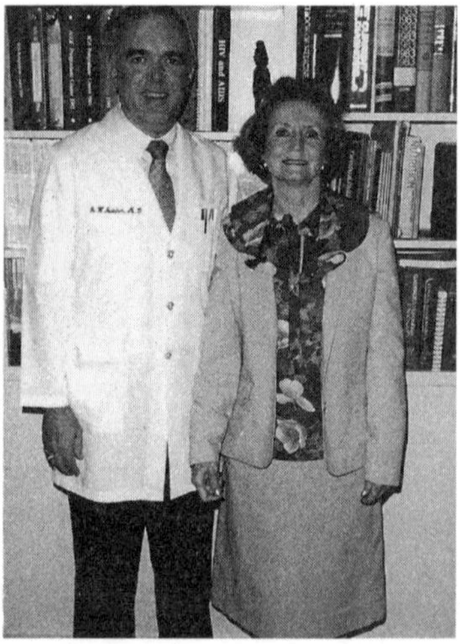

Robert W Swisher MD, West Palm Beach gastroenterologist, diagnosed then treated and saved the life of author Roberta Crawford.

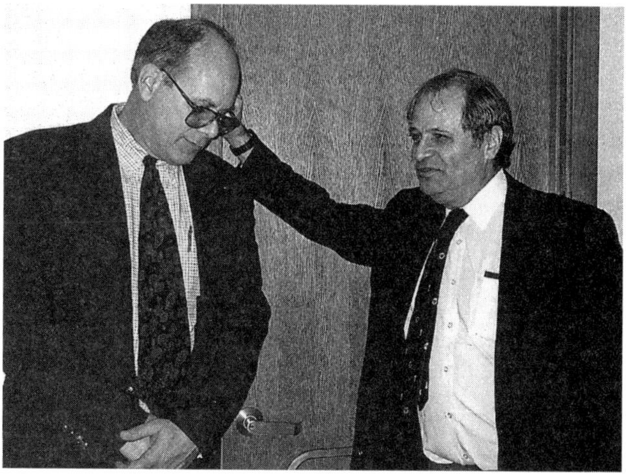

Victor Herbert MD JD, right, hematologist and nutritionist chats at a break during a CDC meeting with James C Barton MD, Birmingham AL hematologist.

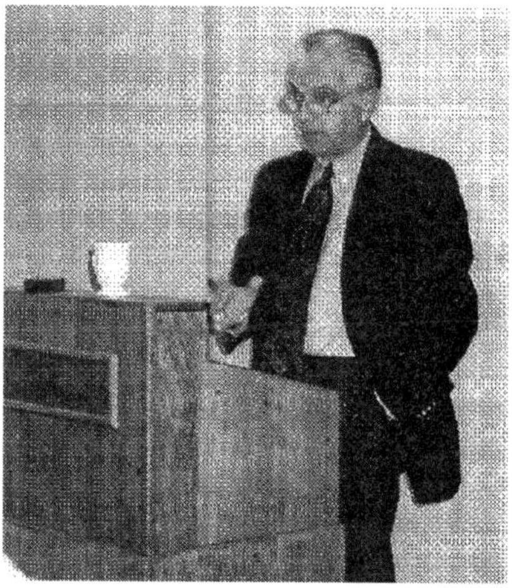

Vincent Felitti MD screens clients for iron at Kaiser Permanente in San Diego.

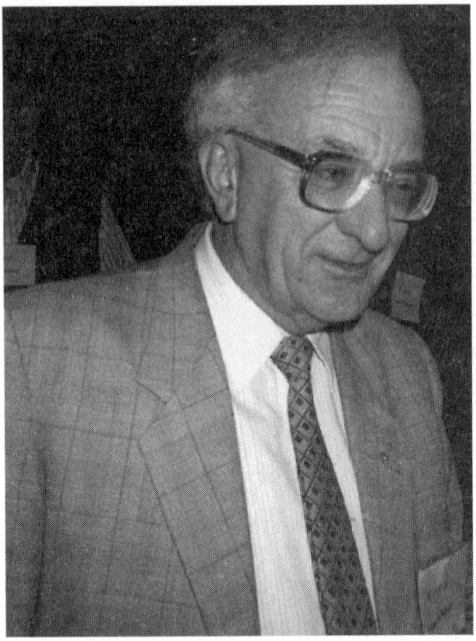

Lawrie Powell MD PhD continues significant studies in Brisbane Australia.

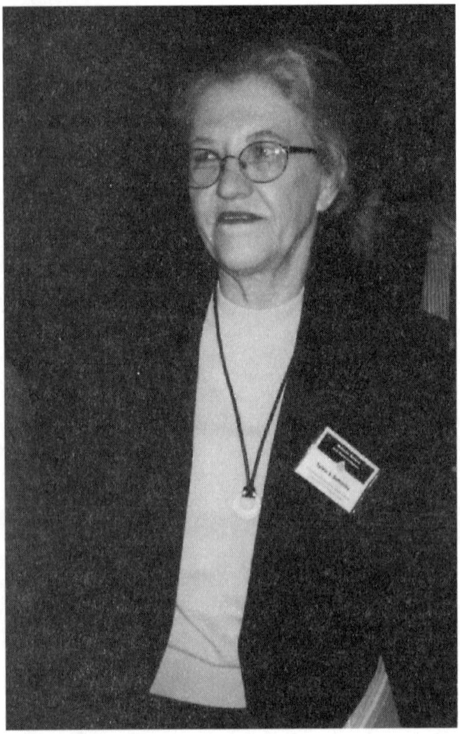

Sylvia Bottomley MD, Professor of Medicine at University of Oklahoma, is noted authority on iron-loading anemia.

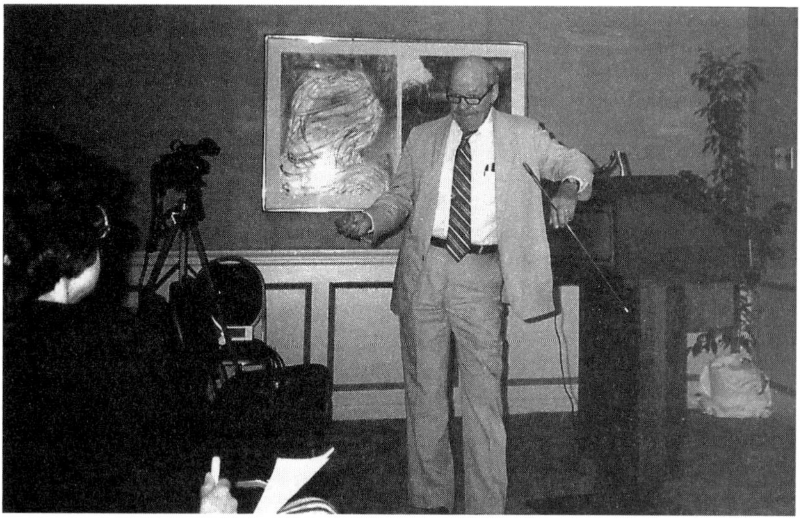

William D Davis MD pioneered treatment of hemochromatosis with WR Arrowsmith in 1950.

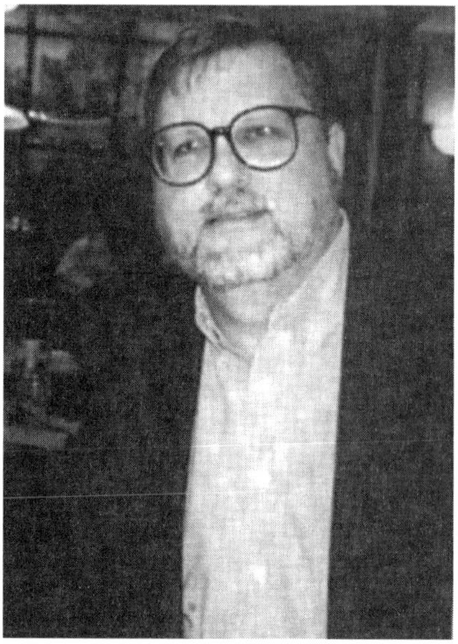

Jerome Sullivan MD PhD pioneered the idea that even a little excess iron can exert damage on *anybody* aside from hemochromatosis. He received an insight while still a medical student.

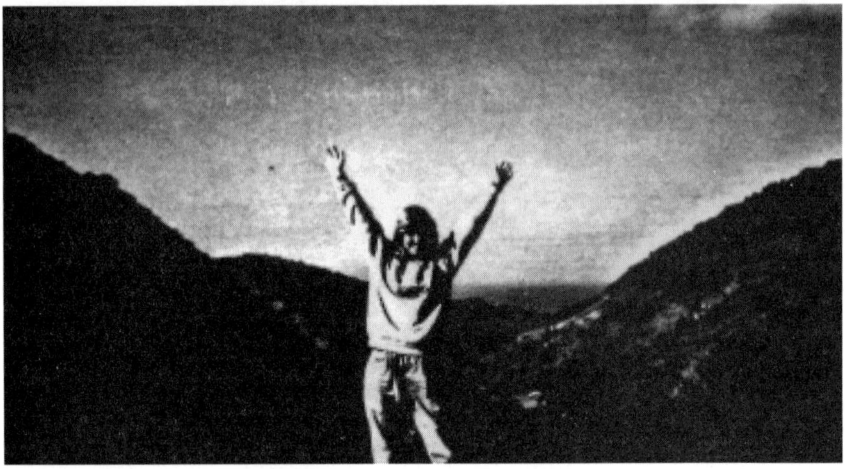

Jennifer Hyland is joyous after intensive treatment to remove iron restores her fertility. She is now mother of an extraordinary little boy.

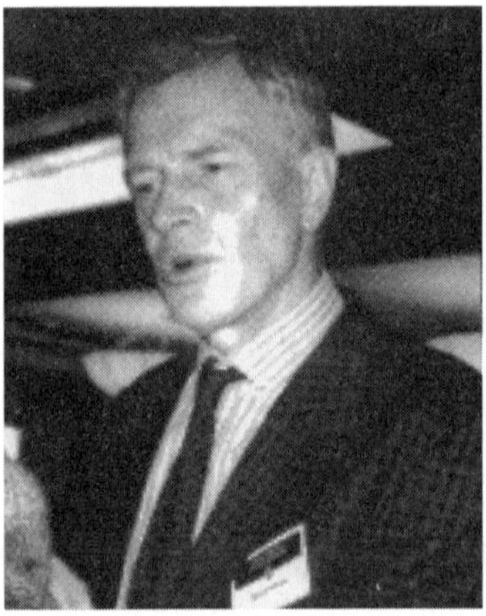

Sigvard Olsen MD, Swedish authority, says, "In Sweden blood banks not only accept blood from individuals with iron overload, but test donors' iron to help identify patients."

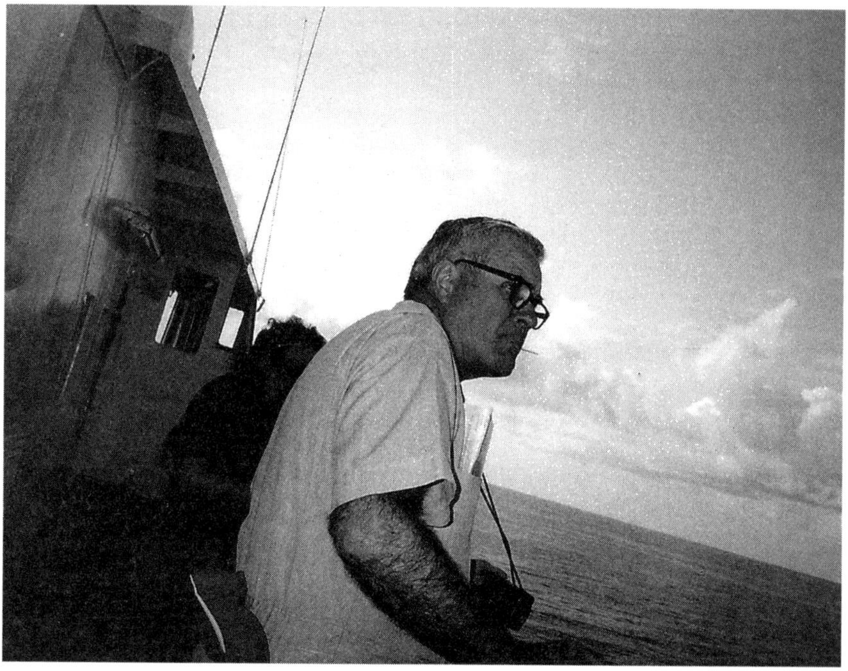

Leslie N Johnston DVM, a veterinarian in Tulsa OK teaches about iron overload in animals and people. He enjoys a cruise following an IOD Symposium in May 1992 in West Palm Beach.

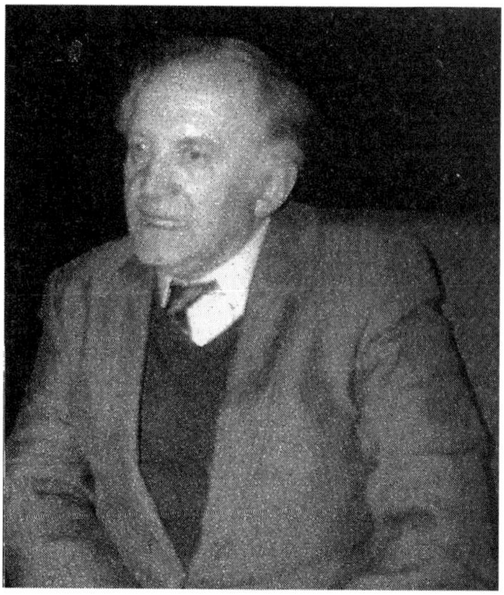

Yuri Tokarev MD of Moscow Russia spoke in 1995 at an IOD Symposium in Rochester NY and later that year invited IOD to participate in an International Symposium on Erythron and Iron in Ryazan Russia.

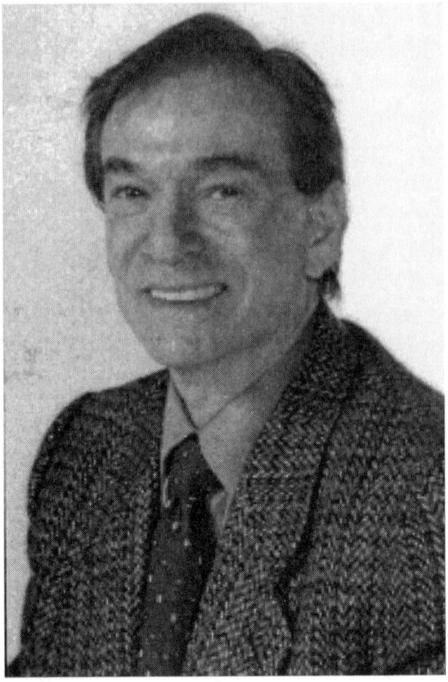

Paul Cutler MD practices in Niagara Falls NY and Canada, studies iron's psychological damage, likes to combine phlebotomy and Desferal chelation to speed iron removal.

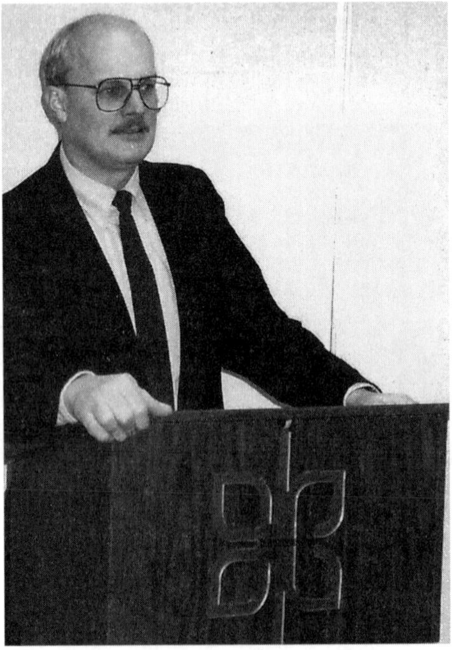

David Witte MD produced Practice Parameters for American College of Pathologists, says, "You can save an entire family."

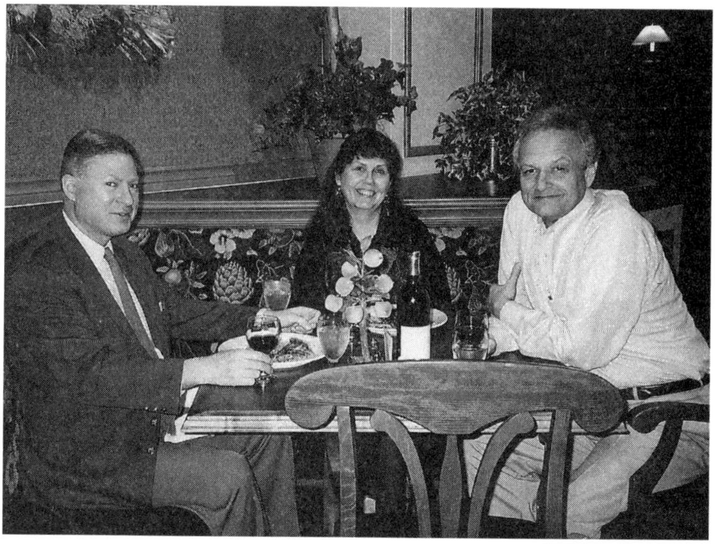

Three iron researchers enjoy dinner in March 1997 at a Centers for Disease Control (CDC) meeting in Atlanta. From the left are Gordon McLaren MD with his wife, Christine McLaren PhD and Gary Brittenham MD.

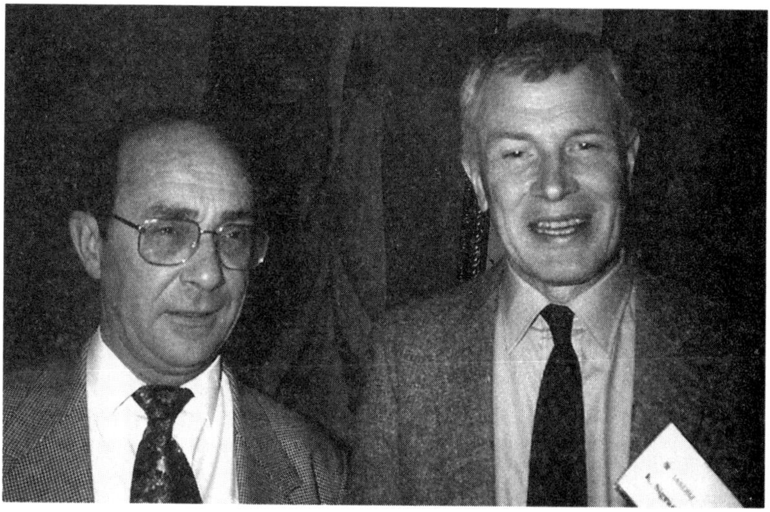

Pierre-Marie Morel, President of Hemochromatose France attends an international biennial meeting in April 1995 in New York. He is taking a break with Sigvard Olsen MD of Sweden.

Table 1

STATE	POPULATION	BOTH GENES	SINGLE GENES
Alabama	4,319,000	21,595	561,470
Alaska	609,000	3,045	79,170
Arizona	4,555,000	22,775	592,150
Arkansas	2,523,000	12,615	327,990
California	32,268,000	161,340	4,194,840
Colorado	3,893,000	19,465	506,090
Connecticut	3,270,000	16,350	425,100
Delaware	732,000	3,630	95,160
Florida	14,654,000	73,270	1 ,905,020
Georgia	7,486,000	37,430	973,180
Hawaii	1,187,000	5,935	154,310
Idaho	1,210,000	6,050	157,300
Illinois	11,886,000	59,430	1,545,180
Indiana	5,864,000	29,320	762,320
Iowa	2,852,000	14,260	370,760
Kansas	2,595,000	12,975	337,350
Kentucky	3,908,000	19,540	508,040
Louisiana	4,352,000	21,760	565,760
Maine	1,242,000	6,210	161,460
Maryland	5,094,000	25,470	662,220
Massachusetts	6,118,000	30,590	795,340
Michigan	9,774,000	48,870	1,279,620
Minnesota	4,686,000	23,430	609,180
Mississippi	2,731,000	13,655	355,030
Missouri	5,402,000	27,010	702,260
Montana	879,000	4,395	114,270
Nebraska	1,657,000	8,285	215,410
Nevada	1,677,000	8,385	218,010
New Hampshire	1,173,000	5,865	152,490
New Jersey	8,053,000	40,265	1,046,890
New Mexico	1,730,000	8,650	224,900
New York	18,137,000	90,685	2,357,810
North Carolina	7,425,000	37,125	965,250
North Dakota	641,000	3,205	83,330

STATE	POPULATION	BOTH GENES	SINGLE GENES
Ohio	11,186,000	55,930	1,454,180
Oklahoma	3,317,000	16,585	431,210
Oregon	3,243,000	16,215	421,590
Pennsylvania	12,020,000	60,100	1,562,600
Rhode Island	967,000	4,835	125,710
South Carolina	3,760,000	8,800	488,800
South Dakota	738,000	3,690	95,940
Tennessee	5,368,000	26,840	697,840
Texas	19,439,000	97,195	2,527,070
Utah	2,059,000	10,295	267,670
Vermont	589,000	2,945	76,570
Virginia	6,734,000	33,670	875,420
Washington	5,610,000	28,050	729,300
West Virginia	1,816,000	9,080	236,080
Wisconsin	5,170,000	25,850	672,100
Wyoming	480,000	2,400	62,400

These gene probabilities are based on the most conservative estimates, that is, one in 200 carries both genes, thirteen percent carries a single gene. The figures do not allow for greater frequence among the Irish or among African-Americans.Population figures are estimates from the U. S. Census Bureau in 1997.

In addition to those genetically affected are an unknown number of non-genetic cases of iron overload.

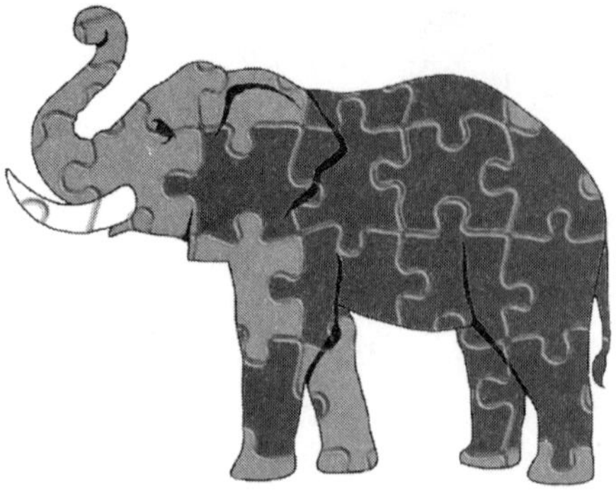

PART 3

If it's so common, why is it misdiagnosed?

Chapter 12

The Cover Up

A moment of silence for the millions whose iron overload was misdiagnosed through many generations. And for those among us whose excess iron is still being neglected.

Let's understand that every doctor wants to make a correct diagnosis. A doctor feels satisfaction in identifying a condition that is treatable and knowing that with treatment the patient is going to improve and feel better. Hemochromatosis is just such a condition, when detected early. Unfortunately many diseases "cover up" the underlying excess iron. These diseases then distract the physician away from the source of the trouble.

During the spring that Rhonda lost her life, Gary, almost 23, in Tomah, Wisconsin, died from a massive hemorrhage. Although an autopsy was performed, hemochromatosis was not diagnosed. Since that time, the diagnosis of his father and two brothers, together with Gary's medical records, have shown the probable true cause of his death.

In the state of Indiana Eric, his brother and his sister were all correctly diagnosed, three out of four siblings. Their father had died in a Veterans Administration hospital of cirrhosis. Eric's doctor suspected that the father had suffered undetected iron overload. Eric secured his father's medical records and made two copies, the second for his other doctor in Florida.

The Florida doctor examined the reports and said, "I see no evidence of hemochromatosis." The first doctor, however, noticed numbers that heightened his suspicions. He asked for the liver slides. When they arrived, they had not been stained to reveal iron so of course no iron was detected. Technicians stained the specimen with Prussian blue, and there it was!

Missed at autopsy? If medical examiners don't suspect iron overload, they don't look for it. If they don't look for iron overload, they can miss it.

Doctors who are alert to hemochromatosis, who look for it in their patients, are increasingly finding it. Often the number of diagnoses surprises the investigating physicians.

James C. Barton, MD, since 1987 has been making a diagnosis almost every week — by looking for it! Dr. Barton is a hematologist at Brookwood Medical Center in Birmingham, Alabama.

A man in a small Florida town became increasingly worried about his seventy-year-old mother. "I took her to twenty doctors," he said, "every doctor in town." None of them thought of iron until the twentieth doctor. By then the patient was dying, dying from advanced hemochromatosis. Iron was found in her pancreas; — that explained the diabetes — in the liver; — that explained the cirrhosis; skin; — it was brown and wrinkled; brain ... kidneys. "She died from liver failure," said her son. For a long time after her death he was obsessed with the disease. "I went around trying to find out something." At that time, the mid-seventies, there was no information available to the general public. "I kept thinking: nineteen doctors!" The man became so worn out with anger that for two years he couldn't talk about it. "Then," he said, "I threw away all her medical records."

In January 1994 I made a list of the Top Ten Reasons that excess iron was neglected for 100 years.

Reason #10. Dollars, dollars and more dollars. Iron is cheap. Iron sits firmly perched on a nutritional pedestal. $1,435 billion is spent retail for multivitamins with minerals and without. You really have to work to find vitamins without iron. Sales of iron alone account for another $20 million. We still call this a modern obscenity. So what's the difficulty? Unlike other poisons, iron is necessary for every body cell, is poisonous only in excess.

Reason #9. Iron tests were not available. In 1925 tests were developed to measure serum iron. The TIBC (Total Iron Binding Capacity) test was developed in 1944. A test for ferritin didn't come along until 1956, and "normal" levels were set far too high. One vital fact was not well known, that once absorbed, iron is not excreted. Daily iron loss is only one to one and a half milligrams. This means that the same amount needs to be replaced: one to one and a half milligrams.

Reason #8. Iron tests are still not being used. Only a few labs such as MetPath, now Quest, offer iron tests routinely. Such labs are then shot down by the U. S. government (Medicare) and sneered at by a television show (*60 MINUTES*). Often the tests are misinterpreted, with low iron reading seen as iron deficiency with little attention paid to the underlying condition. A low iron test points to blood loss from a bleeding ulcer or tumor cells.

Reason #7. Medical intransigence. A better word is *inertia.* Some physicians can't bring themselves to face new knowledge. Louis Pasteur had the same trouble getting them to recognize germs.

Reason #6. Rusty, contaminated information. As late as the 1990s we could still open a prestigious medical journal (JAMA Dec 15 1993 vol 270, No 23) and read the following line: "Although [the Canadian Task Force on the Periodic Health Examination] did recommend *hemoglobin* measurement during pregnancy to identify *iron deficiency...*"

Reason #5. The body damage covers up the iron. Patients with cancer, heart or thyroid disease, chronic fatigue, cirrhosis, diabetes, impotence or arthritis are not being tested for iron values. Which means they are not receiving the most basic care. The symptoms are treated without regard for the underlying cause. The cause may or may not be excess iron, but it only makes sense to rule out the possibility.

Reason #4. Anemia is almost always assumed to be iron deficiency. The U. S. Preventive Services Task Force published a Policy Statement on Routine Iron Supplementation During Pregnancy (JAMA Dec 15 1993). While the paper admits that "There is currently little evidence to suggest that routine iron supplementation during pregnancy is beneficial in improving clinical outcomes for the mother, fetus or newborn," the paper is filled with references to iron deficiency and anemia indiscriminately as if they were identical terms. Iron deficiency is a condition of low iron levels, usually from chronic blood loss or tumor; anemia is a condition of low hemoglobin or red cell lack plus other abnormalities and **can accompany iron overload.** It's dangerous to give iron without knowing iron levels, and when low, knowing the reason.

Reason #3. Families are unwilling to harbor "bad genes." But Paul Steven Miller, speaking at a conference of Alliance of Genetic Support Groups in September 1998 said, "Everybody has a genetic disposition for some abnormality." Where's the disgrace if yours causes you to absorb excess iron? First of all, we now know that everyone should know his iron levels. If someone in the family has been lucky enough to be diagnosed with iron overload, other family members have received an early warning denied to most. Skepticism is fine, but stupidity is ridiculous.

Reason #2. There's no pill to treat it, no way to enrich pharmaceutical companies. In fact, iron overload is a cheap disease to detect and to treat. After this condition receives the attention it deserves, our entire health care system and its economics will improve remarkably.

Reason #1. It's too simple. How can it be right? Find out how much iron you have. If it's a little elevated, become a blood donor and bring down the ferritin. That's all.

Robert Swisher MD, researcher at the VA Medical Center in Riviera Beach, Florida, said, "The inertia is incredible in view of the wealth of documented evidence."

A patient in the Chicago area was told seven years ago that his illness was all mental. He was institutionalized. He was given shock treatments. He was made to believe he was "crazy." Now he receives a correct diagnosis. Now he's really mad.

"Hemochromatosis is the most unrecognized problem in American medicine," said Kenneth Bridges MD of Harvard at a blood bank conference in April 1995 in Boston.

"It seems ironic that still, after so much has been written concerning hemochromatosis," writes Virgil F. Fairbanks, MD, "myths and misconceptions remain widely prevalent." [Hemochromatosis: The Neglected Diagnosis, Mayo Clinic Proceedings April 1986].

One tenacious myth has it that hemochromatosis is a rare disease. The typical physician, if he was exposed to iron overload even briefly in medical school, was told the disease is rare. He believes he will never see a case in practice.

Some professors of medicine continue to write papers, using out-of-date rates of incidence based on the numbers of *recognized* cases in hospitals.

"Is it any wonder," writes William H. Crosby, MD, "that many physicians do not consider it in their differential diagnosis?" [Hemochromatosis, The Missed Diagnosis, Arch Intern Med Vol. 146 June 1986].

Because of the rarity myth, physicians neglect to study it. "They retain misconceptions about its nature, diagnosis and treatment," Crosby said. "The diagnosis of hemochromatosis is easy:" writes Crosby in the same paper, "it requires the demonstration of increased amounts of iron."

The New York Academy of Sciences magazine, The Sciences, May/June 1987, carried a piece, "The Nine Lives of Discredited Data." The piece was critical of the proliferation of textbooks, their slick packaging, commercialization and lessening of scholarship quality. "The repetition in text after text of discredited data," writes Diane B. Paul, "is part of a larger trend —" The author finds textbooks to be less concerned with content. "Indeed, many are virtual clones," she said.

While the same cannot be said of the medical journals, misconceptions about hemochromatosis do flourish through a similar repetition.

However, even more of a block to correct diagnosis is the cover up by the many diseases caused by the underlying excess iron. Too many doctors are treating symptoms and are giving inadequate attention to the cause.

Donald, the young California dentist, looks back over the course of his experience. Hemochromatosis symptoms were obvious: diseased joints with typical abnormalities that were clear on xray; a bronzed complexion; enlarged liver and a lack of serological evidence of arthritis. The doctor "didn't bother to take the simple blood tests to rule out hemochromatosis," Donald said. Early treatment, blood removal to unload iron before body injury, would have prevented much anguish for Donald and his family. Following one hundred twenty phlebotomies, years too late, a total hip replacement and a knee operation, Don became totally disabled at the age of forty-five. All because his doctor was not updated on the signs and symptoms and prevalence of hemochromatosis.

Patients find it incredible that they must pay with their health and lives for this ignorance. Updated information is available to the many practitioners who are taking a serious interest.

It was clear to us that if doctors and the public could be made sufficiently aware, patients would be detected and much suffering could be avoided. IOD began waging campaigns for media attention. In the early nineteen eighties Sandra Thomas joined the organization, and added her enthusiasm to the awareness project. Sandra's mother had received a diagnosis and was being treated. Soon Sandra joined the Board of Directors as Director of Public Education. She hounded newspapers, television stations and radio stations, and managed to get some attention on the subject, a feature story here, a talk show there. The result invariably was a flood of inquiries. However national awareness continued to elude us. It was the same with serious funding. We felt we were chipping through granite, advancing maybe one centimeter a day.

In 1984 IOD conducted a survey of its network of diagnosed patients, then two hundred forty families. The heart-hurting responses revealed a chronicle of delayed diagnoses that resulted in premature deaths, fortunes misspent on useless medical bills and destroyed lives. The wonder was that the patients and their families had suffered so much with such patience and resignation. A high percentage of the cases were plainly legally actionable.

Twenty-five percent of the patients had seen physicians for six to ten years in pursuit of a correct diagnosis, and nineteen percent were misdiagnosed beyond ten years! Although hemochromatosis is among the cheapest of diseases to detect and treat, fifty percent of those surveyed had spent more than $5,000 before being correctly diagnosed. It cost another thirty-two percent of the patients between $1,000 and $5,000.

Ten patients reported financial ruin. An additional fifty-three patients said their dollar cost was "impossible to calculate, but the human loss was even greater." They reported grief and bitterness.

The IOD survey showed also that doctors are prescribing iron for patients who are already dying of iron overload.

Betty, a Milan, Indiana teacher, says that "because of the delay in treatment and a wrong diagnosis," she spent thousands of dollars and finally had to give up her profession.

Kelly, a college student in Raleigh, North Carolina, fervently hopes that awareness will be created, because lack of it cost the life of her father.

Patients write comments to IOD protesting that you have to "be lucky" to receive a correct diagnosis.

"Although I had studied the disease years ago at Mayo Clinic," said a California dermatologist, "I never thought of it as something I myself would have." Suddenly at the age of fifty-one, it dawned on him that what his symptoms added up to was that"obscure" disease, interesting to study — but who would have thought?

What roadblocks stand in the way of correct diagnosis? What causes physicians to veer off down deadend pathways? The IOD survey brought several factors into clear focus.

Roadblock #1. Misconception about the proper place of iron in human health and how to measure body iron.

Somewhere in history we got off the track about iron. Possibly antique dietary habits did cause deficiencies. It is generally accepted even today that populations in "emerging" countries suffer iron deficiency. We must re-examine these beliefs. If iron deficiencies are secondary to parasitic diseases, as is often the case, then it's the parasites that need the attention. Proper tests to measure iron stores have not long been in wide use and are not used as routinely as they should be. If people in "advanced" countries have to be "lucky" to get iron tested, why is it that the millions elsewhere, said to be iron deficient, know their iron levels? Or do they? Isn't their so-called iron deficiency based on hemoglobin levels just as they are too often in the United States? What substantiates the iron deficiency?

The horrible truth is that many doctors mistakenly believe they are measuring iron when they order complete blood counts, hemoglobin, hematocrit. They mistakenly think a low red cell count means a low iron level.

Such ignorance is dangerous for the unlucky patient who suffers from both iron overload and anemia — and there are many such patients.

The literature reports a case of a woman without symptoms whose transferrin saturation was ninety-two percent. The normal range is between twelve and forty-five percent.. However, after being bled for six months her iron status returned to normal. [Gastroenterol 75:886-88, 1978]. The woman may be unaware of her rare good fortune to receive early detection and prompt treatment that prevented damage.

A woman from Sylmar, California wrote to IOD saying she had missed a television program about the organization and she needed information. "My doctor recently found that I have an extremely high level of iron for no apparent reason," she wrote. She did not know what action to take.

An Illinois family grieved for their mother, who died June 24, 1982, only five weeks after the diagnosis. She was sixty-nine. The medical examiner who performed the post-mortem said, "except for the hemochromatosis, she would have lived for many more years."

The woman had thirteen children, and was presumably anemic. Doctors had treated her with Feosol tablets, three times a day, for many years. In 1977 during attempted gall bladder surgery, cirrhosis was discovered. Still no diagnosis. The gall bladder was good. The patient had actually undergone a previous liver biopsy in 1972 during a hysterectomy. At that time it was observed the liver was "enlarged and hobnailed." Said her daughter, Lillian, "My mother

... had maybe one drink a year."

The family became worried as their mother began suffering bouts of pneumonia, loss of memory, swollen feet and arthritis. Her children insisted she see a doctor, but when she finally did go, the doctor said these symptoms were not uncommon in an elderly person.

During the winter of 1981 their mother became too exhausted to dress. She began staying in bed all day. Again her family took her to a doctor. This time tests showed diabetes and "Parkinson's disease." After her release from the hospital, the patient continued on a downward course. Again to the hospital, where — belatedly — hemochromatosis was diagnosed. Now many, many iron tests were given. Now, at the end, two units of blood were removed in an attempt to take away decades of iron accumulation.

"We foolishly believed what the doctor told us," Lillian said. "We are just average people with no medical background." The doctor had kept telling their mother, "You're doing OK. Just stick to your diet and get lots of rest."

In April, 1964, Freda first heard the word: hemochromatosis. "Your husband is a dying man," doctors told her, "It's hemochromatosis." Freda had met her husband in 1934 and was struck by his "startling" color, sallow. He was being treated with vitamin B12 for anemia. He was tired a great deal of the time and needed lots of sleep. During the couple's marriage, Oscar saw several internists. He developed heart disease and began seeing cardiologists. After many years of severe health problems, Oscar suffered the ascites (fluid spilling into the abdominal cavity) of late-stage hemochromatosis. When doctors finally gave a name to Oscar's illness, they told Freda that "no medication is available."

Not long after that in Louisville, Kentucky, another woman, Lidia, watched her husband die. He had been under the care of "many doctors" for ten years. "They couldn't determine what was wrong with him." He eventually was diagnosed and received treatment, but by then he had suffered too much liver damage. Lidia's husband died soon after.

Roadblock #2. Wrong perceptions about the "rarity" of hemochromatosis.

"I've never seen a case in thirty years of practice," the physician told a patient. Thirteen percent of his patients carried at least one gene. If that doctor had treated three thousand patients during his career, he had possibly seen but not recognized fifteen iron overloaded patients. He had not suspected excess iron, he had not looked for it, he had not found it.

"My sister's husband died (from hemochromatosis) at age forty-six," wrote Mary from Dayton, Ohio. The patient's daughter was diagnosed and was successfully treated. Doctors had said her father died of a heart attack. "If the autopsy had not been performed," said Mary, "heaven only knows if she (the daughter) would be alive now."

In Mexico Irene went to the "ten leading doctors in Mexico City," she said. Irene's complaint was large areas of "depigmentation of the skin." She was given the name of a disorder that was considered inconsequential, and told to go home and "be thankful that it was nothing worse."

A doctor in Mazatlan gave her a medicine to rub over a large area of the skin with instructions to sun-bathe. Irene followed the doctor's instructions, suffered second degree burns and spent two weeks in bed healing. After the burns healed, the spots were still there.

Irene and her brother both developed diabetes. Her brother traveled to Mayo Clinic, where his hemochromatosis diagnosis was made. He called his sister at once and told her to have her iron levels tested. Three doctors refused to order the tests, telling her "not to worry." The physician who was treating her for diabetes was one of the three. She insisted, and he finally agreed to the tests. A short time later, her doctor called her at the hotel where she was staying. Yes, the tests did show abnormality; she needed to start treatment immediately.

Irene began an intensive bloodletting program that eventually "de-ironed" her. Later she continued with maintenance phlebotomies of blood removal every three months. Now she says she "feels grand." If her diagnosis was hard to get, at least the treatment was correct. She remembers, however, an uncle who died of diabetes, with other symptoms similar to hers and her brother's.

From the Midwest Richard writes that he is a forty-three-year old black male prisoner who had been treated for "chronic hepatitis" for two years when the prison physician discovered hemochromatosis. If Richard fully realizes how unusually lucky you have to be to receive a correct diagnosis; if he also understands that a correct diagnosis is essential to prevent fatality, Richard may be telling himself it's a case of being in the right place at the right time!

A family in the state of Washington includes a mother, daughter and two sons, all being treated. One son had trouble convincing the military he needed treatment, and the daughter's doctor was also skeptical, although her serum ferritin reached 750. Normal top limit for women is usually considered to be around 150.

Phil and Arlene clicked at first meeting. "He was my knight in shining armor," she says. Right away he confessed to her that he was "disabled," from a car accident. "But," he added, "nobody believes me." Arlene did believe, and she took Phil to her family doctor. The doctor put Phil in the hospital and gave him a "complete physical." He found nothing wrong. Ten more doctors "found nothing wrong."

Then the couple was lucky enough to see a doctor who made the diagnosis of hemochromatosis. During those years a helpful pharmacist had suggested a food supplement that contained plenty of iron. "It's loaded with vitamins and iron," he said, "which can't hurt." The doctor who made the diagnosis had sent Phil's blood work to MetPath,now Quest, a New Jersey lab with branches throughout the country, that routinely adds iron tests. IOD recommends that all labs add these tests, and that doctors and hospitals order them as a screening precaution.

Roadblock #3. Wrong criteria for diagnosis.

Medical texts describe hemochromatosis as a condition that requires myocardial disease, arrhythmia, congestive heart failure, sterility and impotence, debilitating arthritis, lethargy, skin pigmentation and diabetes. All of those misfortunes can happen, but they need not.

Lack of awareness leads some physicians to wait until the patient has developed this full-blown picture before beginning treatment. The physician may want to wait for the complications, but the patient would rather not. Logic demands that if excess iron is present, it must be removed. And while we're about it, let's re-examine how much is too much. If you don't want to call it hemochromatosis, call it iron overload. Call it too much iron. Call it anything, just get rid of it.

Louise of Highland Park, Illinois, lost her husband in 1984. "His doctor kept insisting that he stop drinking," she wrote, "but John never did drink much. He could not persuade the doctor that his liver problem had some other basis." Louise can't understand why her husband had to die. "I find it hard to believe that so many physicians had so much trouble pinpointing it."

Roadblock #4. The many diseases that cover up the causative iron.

When a physician makes a diagnosis of diabetes or cirrhosis or arthritis, he or she thinks the diagnosis has been made. How often will doctors wonder "what caused the diabetes?" It is perfectly true that any of these diseases can occur without the involvement of iron. However, when iron is the underlying factor, no amount of testing, no method of treatment will do the patient any lasting good unless the iron is removed.

Excessive iron may be lurking unrecognized in the patient with arthritis, hypothyroidism, cardiomyopathy, diabetes, impotence, sterility or cirrhosis. If the causative iron is unmasked in time and removed, some of the body injury may be reversible.

Joan, a sixty-nine-year-old Wyoming woman received a belated diagnosis in 1983. For twelve years doctors had kept telling her that her iron levels were elevated and that liver function tests showed abnormality. It was a case of "Let's wait and see what happens." Two years before the diagnosis, Joan did undergo a liver biopsy. The gastroenterologist told her that liver cells were normal, that there was iron in the liver, but because the cells were normal, it was not hemochromatosis. That was the first time she heard that strange word.

After moving to Tulsa and starting with a new doctor, Joan insisted on iron tests. By then her serum ferritin was 558. Joan had previously had a hysterectomy, a common history of iron overloaded patients. She was fifty-two at the time. Because of heavy bleeding caused by the fibroid tumor that led to the operation, her hemoglobin dropped to nine, and Joan was medicated with iron. The schedule of medication lasted for years.

Cathy, an Orlando woman, became greatly concerned after her gynecologist told her she suffered "probable hemochromatosis." Nothing was said about where to go from there. Cathy was uncertain what her next step should be, until she happened to read a feature story reprinted from the Chicago Tribune, written by Stevenson Swanson.

There's no doubt that such newspaper and magazine coverage has directly saved lives. A previous excellent piece by Jeffrey Weiss in The Miami Herald was reprinted in many Knight-Ridder papers and pointed the way to correct diagnosis for hundreds of patients who had been awash in ignorance and confusion.

Roadblock #5. The treating of symptoms.

Doctors are busy, pressured. They do not like to turn away patients, and their case loads may be excessive.

I took my mother to a hematologist in Tampa, Florida. A kind, friendly man, he questioned her. "I sometimes get dizzy," she said. "Well, I can give you something for that," was his reply. That kind of response is unsatisfactory. The patient doesn't want "something" for the dizziness. She mentions it in hopes of learning *why*. She has been uneasily wondering about the problem during the long wait between doctor appointments. Does dizziness indicate a need for further investigation?

It's too much to expect this kind of careful evaluation from every doctor for every patient. But I do want it for my mother, don't I? Perhaps *dizziness is* too nonspecific, too elusive to pin down. But doctors are over-quick to reach for their prescription pads. God knows they write too many prescriptions for iron.

What it boils down to is the competence of the individual doctor. The patient searching for a correct diagnosis can go to the most prestigious clinic in the land and be misdiagnosed. He can go to the most brilliant physician and be misdiagnosed.

A country doctor who understands iron, a medical student still in school who understands iron, would be a safer bet, if you hope for an early diagnosis of iron overload.

The information gap — along with the wide dissemination of misinformation — is the single greatest problem of hemochromatosis and other iron overload diseases. There would hardly be a problem at all if correct information could lead patients and their physicians to early detection followed by adequate treatment.

The medical ignorance is scandalous. IOD has persevered for more than two decades to create awareness. Yes, there has been progress. But substantial financial help was hard to come by.

Workers have been using a teaspoon to fill a Grand Canyon of abysmal ignorance.

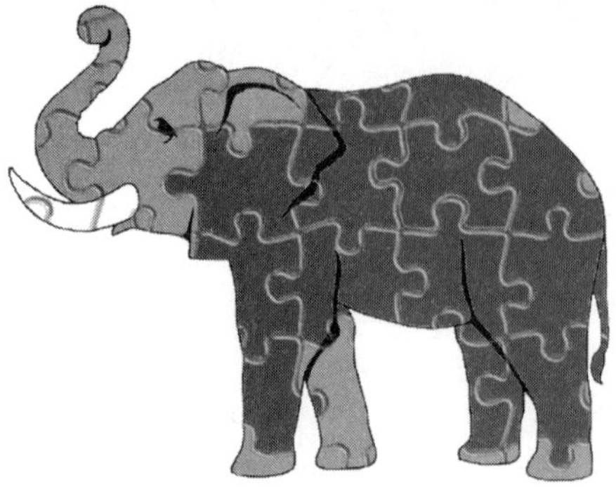

Part 4

"How in the world do you get it?"

Chapter 13

Your Genes Give It To You

If your genes are one hundred percent "normal," you are altogether perfect. If so, you are indeed rare, since perfection is a rarity, isn't it? People working on the Genome Project have said that everyone has about seven abnormal genes or mutations. Suppose you have an abnormality for iron metabolism. Only a slight defect can have a disastrous consequence. *If you neglect it.*

Writing in **IRONIC BLOOD** (Vol.4 No.4), William H. Crosby, MD, said, "A key concept to the understanding of normal iron metabolism is balance; e.g. when iron moves out of the body a corresponding quantity must move in to maintain balance. When old red blood cells — together with their iron — are removed from the blood, a like number must replace them. This is true of all cell populations that are continually replaced.

"The total body burden of iron in a normal adult is about four grams (gm) or four thousand milligrams (mg). About one-half is invested in the hemoglobin of red blood cells. Somewhat less than one-third is storage iron that has no function except as a reserve. The rest is spread across all the other cells of the body. Every cell requires some iron."

Crosby explains that every cell in the body has to have iron. This includes cancer cells. It also includes bacteria. We need only a minute amount, which we get from food. "Our American diet provides each day ten to twenty mg of food iron," Crosby wrote. "The normal person absorbs what he needs of this and the remainder is defecated. He absorbs just enough to replace what has been lost. With other nutrient metals — calcium, sodium, zinc, etc. — random quantities are absorbed; what is not required is excreted. Iron is different. Once absorbed, there is no excretory mechanism of iron. When unneeded iron enters the body it must be added to the iron stores. The absence of an excretory system does not mean that iron cannot be lost. We shed cells continually from the surfaces of our body; the skin, the intestine, the urinary tract. Every cell contains some iron. The cumulative loss of all the detritus amounts to about one mg per day." Think of that. Only one milligram of iron is needed to replace daily loss. For the sake of our good health we must see iron in a new light. A little goes a long way. There is another method of losing iron, though, as Crosby pointed out a few years ago. "We also can lose iron by bleeding. The red blood cell contains much more iron than any other; one gram of red cells contains one milligram of iron. The loss of blood is a prodigal wasting of iron. This is the basis for treating hemochromatosis by removal of blood (phlebotomy)." Bloodletting conjures scenes of ancient medical practices, but it turns out the ancients may have been onto something. The procedure is now proving to be a life saver.
Your body will protect you from excess iron if your iron metabolism is operating normally.

"Because excess iron cannot be excreted," Crosby writes, "the body's iron balance is maintained by limiting the amount that is absorbed. Just enough is absorbed to offset what is lost, one mg per day in shed skin cells, etc. When in addition, blood is lost, causing an iron deficiency of some degree, the intestine modifies its avidity and absorbs more iron from the diet, attempting to maintain the balance. When the deficit is corrected, the intestine reasserts its ability to keep out the dietary iron that is not needed. The normal absorptive intestine behaves in an intelligent way, responding with precision to the body's requirement for iron.

"An important function of the small intestine is its ability to refrain from absorbing available dietary iron that the body does not need. Remember: the ability to refrain from absorbing available dietary iron that the body does not need.

"I emphasize this point because the absence of that ability is the cause of hemochromatosis. Unneeded iron is not kept out. It is absorbed; it cannot be excreted; it must be stored; the storage organs are eventually damaged."

In other words, your iron rejecting mechanism must be doing its job. You must be able to rely on that rejection for protection against iron overload.

"Iron has a great potential for biological activity. When not properly controlled, iron can cause biological damage. It is a poison. In all biologic systems iron is carefully controlled, usually by combining it with a protein.

"Hemoglobin in mammals is the outstanding example. In this compound the protein globin contains iron that is locked into a pigment ring, heme. Hemoglobin iron combines easily and reversibly with oxygen in the lungs and releases it where it is needed in the body."

If cancer cells are forming, they consume some of the iron, removing it from circulation. This is why you must investigate for a possible malignancy when your iron tests show a true iron deficiency. There is no medical logic in responding to iron deficiency by iron medication without first checking into the reason.

"Iron must be moved from place to place, from the spleen where red cells are destroyed to the marrow where new red cells are formed. The same iron atoms are used over and over again in successive generations of red cells. When iron may not be needed at the moment, it is placed in storage."

Red cells die and release their iron, which is as good as new. This iron is then recycled into the hemoglobin of red cells.

"The plasma has a specific iron-binding protein, transferrin, that holds and controls iron in transit, picking it up and dropping it off in response to local surfeit or need. The concentration of iron in plasma is about one hundred micrograms per one deciliter. The range of normal values of plasma iron is around fifty to one hundred sixty. The plasma contains enough transferrin to combine with about three hundred micrograms of iron per deciliter. This is the Total Iron Binding Capacity (TIBC). When the concentration of iron is one hundred micrograms, the transferrin is about one-third saturation. This is a normal saturation index (SI). It may be higher or lower and still be normal; it is conventional to regard as abnormal SI below fifteen percent and above fifty percent. People with hemochromatosis have high SI." Note: newer information says the range should be twelve to forty-five percent. As time goes on, this range may again be down-sized.

There was a world-wide race to discover the gene that lasted for years. In August 1996 researchers in Menlo Park, California, announced they had identified the gene responsible for hemochromatosis. Mercator Genetics theorized that a large percentage of these patients may be descended from a single individual. That person contributed the DNA mutation plus ancient surrounding DNA. The gene searchers studied 178 patients.

Labs soon began offering the DNA tests. Confusion abounded. Ernest Beutler MD wrote that "It is unfortunate that the role of 187G mutation has been misinterpreted by several of the leading groups." He said, "They have mistakenly concluded that it is an unrelated polymorphism because they have failed to take into account the fact that it is in complete linkage repulsion from the 845A mutation."

One lab returned a report to a patient, saying she is a "compound heterozygote." The lab found one copy of the C282Y mutation and one copy of the H63D allele.

At that time it was thought that those mutations discovered would identify about 85 percent of affected individuals. Scripps Research Institute put out information that described a high proportion of patients who carry 845A/845A genotype. They are compound homozygotes. Other homozygotes, those with 845G/845G may or may not have the most common form of iron storage.

To complicate matters there are those with single mutations, 845G/845A, heterozygous, or even homozygous with 187C/187C. Most of those with these mutations may not have the iron loading defect, but anyone with the 845 mutation is considered a carrier, that is, a heterozygote in genetics parlance. Other mutations being considered are 187C/187G. Scripps advised such individuals should monitor iron levels. Well, we say that to everybody. There are still mutations to be discovered. And remember, gene or no gene, everyone could overwhelm his body with iron.

The abnormality that disturbs your iron metabolism, that interferes with your normal rejecting ability, comes about through a genetic defect. It is one of the most common disease-causing genetic defects we know about.

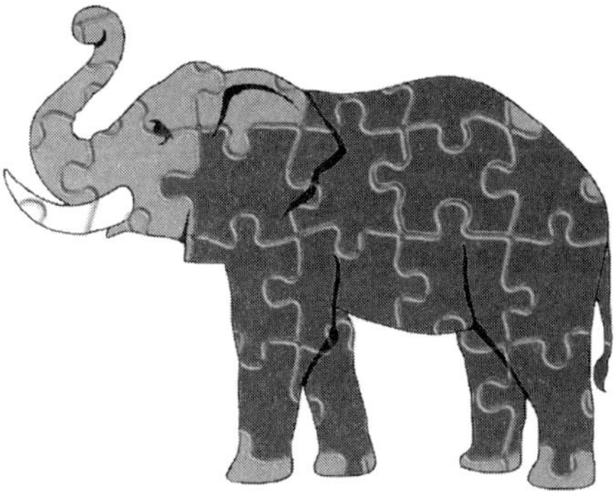

Chapter 14

The Genetic Lottery

Secrets stored by our genes, that are being unraveled, are turning out to be even more exciting than our adventures in space. How marvelous that one set of chromosomes in one cell holds all the plans for the entire body. The sperm cell and egg cell contain chromosome pairs that divide and re-unite, combining into a new individual.

Which genes combine from the mother and which from the father is a toss-up, a genetic roulette. If the spin of the gene wheel tosses you a gene for hemochromatosis, your medical fate could be sealed before you take your first breath. But not necessarily! Not if you recognize the anomaly. Most individuals with such a toss will have plenty of time to protect themselves from iron accumulation. You might ask yourself if you'd rather have a different, less treatable defect. Whether the gene destroys your health or whether you retain your well being depends on your own awareness.

We have partially identified the hemochromatosis gene. Most researchers believe there are others not yet found. In 1975 Marcel Simon, MD, announced the discovery that hemochromatosis patients possess an HLA-A3 gene product much more frequently than do those in the general population. Many scientists throughout the world have confirmed Simon's finding. For decades families were studied to find homozygotes based on matching HLA to the index patient. Unfortunately there were labs that made money offering the HLA to individual patients. There was no valid way to say if you have the HLA-A3 or B14 you have the gene. Only if you matched a family member already diagnosed. And the HLA could be entirely different.

HLA is an abbreviation for histocompatibility locus antigen. These antigens are found on the surface of all human cells. For classification, the antigens have been assigned letter-number designations. Family members who have markers that are identical to those of the patient are considered to be homozygous for the disease. If you are homozygous, you have inherited the double genes. Homozygotes should always be evaluated clinically to determine iron levels. All blood relatives of the patient need careful testing. HLA matching is used as a research tool, and is not a screening procedure.Corwin Q. Edwards, MD, and his colleagues at University of Utah studied a family in which the father was a heterozygote (or single gene carrier) for hemochromatosis. His chart read HLA A2, B13, and A11, B27. The mother was also a single gene carrier, with HLA A29, B44 and A2, B7. Three of their children were homozygotes. Two had identical HLA type A2, B13 and A29, B44. The third surprisingly had A2, B13 and A2, B44. Her HLA type was different from the other homozygotes among her siblings, a finding explained as "recombination." This was the first reported recombination in an individual with hemochromatosis, as reported in *American Journal of Human Genetics, 38:805-811, 1986.* The father's age was forty-eight, the mother forty-six, an affected son eighteen and the two daughters were twenty-one and twelve.

The information yielded to the researchers by this recombination was that it permits "probably assignment of the hemochromatosis allele to the region between HLA-B and HLA-A locations. You could think of the allele as a vehicle for the gene or genes. There are possibly several related genes involved. We had believed that life would be much simpler when we were able to identify the genes. We still believe that life will be a song after we learn how to get into the gene and correct it.

Christopher F. Bryan, PhD, described the genetics of hemochromatosis in *Ironic Blood* (Vol. 3 No. 2). Bryan also presented a new marker for the disease at IOD's Second Symposium. He first became interested in this research while working with Maria de Sousa, MD, PhD, at Sloan-Kettering Institute. Later he continued the studies at Louisiana State University Medical Center in New Orleans. He described his work. "We take normal blood from an individual and mix the cells with sheep red blood cells (RBC) and test at four degrees centigrade. One characteristic of T lymphocytes is that they will bind with sheep RBC. Only T cells do that, not B cells, not monocytes. It's a specific marker for T lymphocytes. It is used throughout the world to identify a sub-population of lymphocyte." Lymphocytes are white blood corpuscles. Bryan described his laboratory work. "If you raise that temperature in this assay to 37 degrees these T lymphocytes will turn loose of those RBC — that occurs in normal individuals. In normal individuals if you take ten lymphocytes and mix them with the sheep RBC you get about one out of ten — about ten percent that form thermostable erythrocyte rosettes." He was talking about red blood cells that formed into shapes of rosettes at a given temperature. "But if you take ten lymphocytes from a hemochromatosis patient four of the cells will form rosettes. Our objective was to characterize that abnormality." Normal red cells form the rosettes in one out of ten cases; red cells from hemochromatosis patients formed the rosettes in four out of ten cases. It is significant that iron was not a factor. In these studies, the iron levels did not influence the number of rosettes, only the genetic material. Let's project a survey of diagnosed patients in IOD's network onto a much larger screen. We can estimate the age groups of those patients in the population who are still undiagnosed.

For example, in a few more than one thousand patients, surveyed in 1988, those at either end of the age scale numbered two in their eighties and two newborn.

We then project onto the estimated one million plus in the United States who are genetically affected, and we arrive at two thousand people in their ninth decade and two thousand newborns likely to suffer end-stage iron overload.

The genetic frequency is estimated at one in two hundred homozygotes and about one in eight heterozygotes. Therefore many more than two thousand newborns are carriers of the genes.

In neonatal hemochromatosis though, the infants are so iron-ridden they may never leave the hospital. It's possible that here too there is a variety of degrees. It seems likely that some older babies with unexplained sudden death could have suffered undetected iron overload. Detection requires suspicion. Someone has to think iron. The younger the patient, the less likely that iron would be suspected.

During the recent past it was believed that the young were rarely affected and children were not even considered. Now that doctors are looking for iron, they are finding it in people formerly thought to be exempt: women, young women, children, babies, the not yet born (fetuses).

Published population figures for the United States and for each of the fifty states can help us estimate the number of people who have both H genes and the number of single gene carriers. See the population chart with photographs in the center of the book. The U. S. population is estimated at close to 270 million. Taking the middle road estimate between the French and Australian studies — the Utah estimate of five per thousand with double H genes and thirteen percent of the population with the single gene — we find that 1,500,000 Americans carry both H genes.

That does not mean that all of these people are suffering the effects of hemochromatosis. Many may be storing iron at normal levels. Remember, though, that Jerome L. Sullivan, MD, PhD, and others suggest that our "normal" perception of iron may be set too high. Additionally, patients' relatives who tested "normal" at one time have sometimes proved to have a considerable iron load at a later examination.

Keep in mind too the variable rate of iron accumulation. A Wisconsin man stored enough iron that it ended his life at twenty-three, while his father was diagnosed only later and is responding to treatment.

A New Jersey man is being treated following the deaths of two sons who died shortly after birth of neonatal hemochromatosis.

Some double gene carriers may not be affected until later decades, or others not at all, as some experts believe.

That brings us to those with single genes. In the U. S. the estimate is about forty-two million. Experts are divided regarding whether this group is at risk for disease. Many authorities say, yes, single gene carriers can develop hemochromatosis by overmedicating with iron.

Victor Herbert MD, JD, says that if you carry the single gene and if you take over the counter vitamin C or iron or abuse alcohol, it's the same as if you had both genes.

Do these people know they are carrying the gene? Almost never. Have they ever heard of the dangers of too much iron? Probably not. Have they heard about iron deficiency? Plenty, thanks to advertising and cereal boxes. Do they get tired? Do they need energy?

Do you think they'll go to the drug store and buy iron supplements? Possibly mega-doses? And if those don't work, perhaps increase the intake?

We can allow that a certain number of single gene carriers will also develop hemochromatosis. That makes substantially more than one million Americans who need to monitor — and drastically lower — their iron levels.

Beyond genes is the simple possibility that *anyone* can overwhelm his body with massive iron intake. Ernest Beutler, MD, wrote, "The evidence inclines us to the view that iron overload by either transfusion or oral iron does lead to hemochromatosis." *[Clinical Disorders of Iron Metabolism. Grune & Stratton, NY 1963].* Even before 1963 it had been firmly established that prolonged transfusional therapy does lead to a fatal overloading of iron unless a chelation drug is used to bind with some of the iron and move it out as waste.

From Pharmacy International, Dec. 1984, comes a story reprinted from Elsevier Publishers BV Amsterdam.

A patient consulted her doctor, presenting a history of weight loss and decreased appetite. Twenty years previously she had been given ferrous sulfate following surgery for prolapsed uterus. Since that time she had continued with the iron medication, which was available at her pharmacy.

The medical report described a frail and wasted woman with grayish complexion. Her transferrin saturation level was more than 88 percent (normal: 12 to 45) and serum ferritin was 8,567 (normal: well under150).

The article says, "Normally iron metabolism is regulated mainly by iron absorption — the regulatory mechanism residing in the mucosal cells of the duodenum and jejunum — however, iron overload may result if the intake of iron is sufficient to overcome this mucosal block." The reference cited was Lawrie W. Powell, MD, PhD, writing in *Haemochromatosis and Related Iron Storage Disease in Liver and Biliary Diseases (W. B. Saunders, Philadelphia, 1979).*

We can assume there is considerable variability in the rate of accumulation. We believe this because a woman in New Jersey can stay alive into her eighties while gradually adding to iron stores year by year. Yet a South Carolina woman accumulates her iron burden so rapidly that she dies at thirty-one.

A New York woman is diagnosed at fifty. She was medicated with iron for twenty years, while an Alabama girl who never took iron dies at twenty-three.

Hemochromatosis may not be only one disease, but, as Crosby has written, "a constellation of diseases."

Erik Bjorn-Rasmussen, MD, made a study of iron metabolism rates at Karolinska Institute in Stockholm. He wrote, "In patients with hereditary haemochromatosis (HH) abnormal functional properties of the macrophage system have been observed." The macrophages he spoke of are the cells that try to fight off infection by engulfing or eating foreign matter. "The present study is a preliminary report of increased transferrin receptor expression on monocytes from twelve patients with HH." A monocyte is a certain type of macrophage. In the twelve patients the monocytes increased their reception of transferrin, a blood component that transports iron around the body. "There was no correlation between the degree of iron overload and the transferrin receptor expression on the monocytes. The results obtained thus indicate that the observed increase in transferrin receptors is not a secondary phenomenon due to systemic iron overload but could be an expression of a primary inborn error of metabolism in HH. The functional aspects of the receptors were not evaluated as they were analyzed by means of monoclonal technique." [Scan J Haematol 1985;34:308-311].

The hapless patient who shows up at his doctor's office with a low blood count is in danger of receiving a prescription for iron. Iron prescriptions are among the most numerous seen by pharmacies. I am glad to say this trend appears to be lessening.

One popular product of the 1950s, 1960s and 1970s was Trinsicon, manufactured by Eli Lilly. "Trinsicon was among the two hundred most prescribed drugs in the U. S. in 1967, a statistic that is likely to make teachers of hematology shudder," said Richard Burack, MC, in The New Handbook of Prescription Drugs (1967).

A special problem with Trinsicon is that in addition to the iron, it also contains a handful of various vitamins, including vitamin C to enhance iron's absorption. If you do respond to the medication, you will not know which of the vitamins is helping. Worse, you will not know that the iron is not contributing to improvement, but instead is being added to stores. Unless of course your iron rejecting mechanism is working to prevent absorption. In that case, it's just iron going down the drain.

If you are among the thirteen out of one hundred people who are carriers of the single gene, medicinal iron could be dangerous for you.

"It cannot be stressed too strongly that iron deficiency is the only disorder that responds to oral iron administration," wrote the authors of "Clinical Disorders of Iron Metabolism" (Ernest Beutler, MD, Virgil F. Fairbanks, MD and John L. Fahey, MD, Grune & Stratton, NY and London, 2nd Ed. 1971). The administration of iron to patients with pernicious anemia, acute or chronic hemolytic anemias, the anemia of chronic renal disease, the anemia of acute infection, the anemia of cancer or any other anemias can do no good, may cause harm, and cannot be condemned too strongly," said the authors. "...the physician is fundamentally obliged to seek site of blood loss." The authors criticized a paper by H. H. Pote, on "Sustained Release Iron Therapy" in Internat. Rec. Med. 171:87-90, 1958. Pote said: "A daily dose of 150 mg of ... ferrous sulfate given in sustained release form will produce adequate hemoglobin response in most patients with hypochromic anemias. This dosage can also provide maintenance therapy for patients with pernicious anemia." The authors commented, "An astonishing statement to have been published in 1958!"

IOD's members were still in 1987 reporting iron medications being given for anemias whose deficiencies were unrelated to iron. They were usually B vitamin deficiencies. One physician was administering Trinsicon to a patient who presumably suffered from pernicious anemia (never differentiated). When the patient questioned why the medicine was not giving enough improvement, the doctor replied that his own mother was being treated in the same way for her "pernicious anemia."

Lynn B. Bailey, PhD, RD, made a study of the folic acid status of teenagers. She found that fifty percent of the youngsters revealed folic acid concentrations "below accepted norms." *[Journal of the American Dietetic Association, Vol 84 No. 7 Jul 1984].* Researchers found that more low income teens were deficient in folic acid than in iron. Iron deficiency was found in twelve percent of the females and in two percent of the males. Folic acid deficiency was found in forty-five percent with less than six ng/ml and fifteen percent were below three ng/ml. [Am J Clin Nutr 35: May 1982, 1023-1032].

Within the same low income areas, the elderly also tested with a large percentage of folic acid deficiency, but with *normal iron levels. [Am J Clin Nutr 1979; 32:2346-53].*

When any of these people are found to have low red cell count or hemoglobin concentration, how are their physicians going to respond?They may or may not carry one of the genes. It doesn't matter. The genes don't kill. It's the iron that kills.

Patients who require a prolonged schedule of blood transfusions for refractory anemia will ultimately acquire a deadly burden of iron, which accumulates and goes into storage in the liver and other organs. The iron then rots out this tissue.

Every patient who requires transfusion therapy for an extended time, and certainly every physician ordering the therapy, should completely understand the consequences: that the large numbers of blood transfusions will result in iron overload. Chelators administered by pump will help slow down accumulation and prolong the patient's life. The chelating agents bind with some of the iron and move it out through the kidneys.

Dot, a woman in a small Georgia town, suffered a severe anemia that required frequent blood transfusions to keep her alive. Her hemoglobin dropped periodically to as low as seven. Her particular anemia was pyridoxine-responsive, but before the vitamin B6 deficiency was discovered, Dot had been given iron, lots of it. Giving iron willy nilly for low hemoglobin was virtually a routine medical practice during most of the decades of the Twentieth Century. The wreckage from this practice is still with us.

Dot required transfusions in addition to pyridoxine. Frequent transfusional therapy, however, brought its own problems. While transfusions were relieving the anemia, the burden of iron eventually became the killer. Dot died of hemochromatosis.

Whether Dot carried any of the genes was not known. However, it is thought that iron-loading anemias are probably associated with at least the carrier state.

Tired? Rundown? Maybe your trouble is iron rich blood instead of "iron poor blood." When you go to a drug store to buy iron medication, warning bells ought to ring.

Your food supply is already giving work to your iron rejecting mechanism. I trust your rejecting mechanism is doing its job and turning away excess iron. But do you know the details of your genetic makeup? The efficiency of your iron metabolism?

William R. Bacon, Mill Valley, California, pharmacist, has sold plenty of iron to customers. Then Bacon was himself diagnosed with hemochromatosis, and he looked at iron with new eyes. "I wonder how many victims of hemochromatosis I have sold dangerous and unnecessary iron supplements," he wrote in *American Pharmacy, Sept. 1984.* Bacon felt he was lucky to be diagnosed. "According to actuarial averages, without treatment I would have died three years ago," he said. "But vigorous treatment saved my life."

Before his diagnosis Bacon had considered iron deficiency to be a common problem with a simple solution. "It all looks much different to me now," he said. "Iron, I have found, deserves more care and caution." In his article Bacon asked his colleagues to "think twice about iron."

In a situation of true iron deficiency, determined by proper evaluation of stores, you'd want to find and correct the internal bleeding, infection or cancer. Just making up the deficit without investigation, would be the same as sedating a watch dog while a thief makes off with the jewels.

A Muncie, Indiana, woman was anemic. Her blood counts were down, and she was iron deficient. Her doctor began transfusing her. Month after month the transfusions continued, but the woman could not seem to maintain a normal hemoglobin.

The patient's husband became worried and he took her to another doctor, who promptly found a source of internal bleeding. The action of the first doctor had been like pouring blood through a sieve.

Iron deficiency requires careful attention, the kind of attention you would pay to a fire alarm or a wildly barking dog in the night.

Most authorities would agree that patients who develop hemochromatosis after overmedication must be carriers of at least the single gene. We'll learn the answers after more research. Meanwhile, consider this. About two thousand American children die every year as a result of consuming a bottle of iron pills. Iron poisoning. The lethal dose of ferrous sulfate for a two-year-old child is approximately three grams; for adults, it ranges from 200 to 250 milligrams per kilogram of body weight. [Victor Herbert, MD, JD, Editor, Mount Sinai School of Medicine Complete Book of Nutrition, St. Martin's Press, 1990]. It has been reported that 100 grams of supplemental iron (ferrous sulfate) can produce mild liver damage.

Whether you do or do not have one of the identified or as yet unidentified genes, dietary iron *can* lead to hemochromatosis. The most famous examples are the black people of the Bantu group of South Africa. They brew alcoholic beverages in iron pots, and get huge quantities of iron leached from the containers. In addition, studies show that alcohol enhances iron absorption.

Genetic studies are just starting among the Bantu-speaking people. This valuable research project needs to be done, but it is believed that many cases of hemochromatosis among the South Africans are acquired and not inherited. Because these genes are so amazingly common I suspect that yes, Bantus carry genes that load iron.

In early stages the iron is distributed differently, but at a certain level, the disease runs a similar course, whether inherited or acquired, and whether acquired by transfusional, medicinal or dietary means.

For too long iron has occupied a high position on the nutritional pedestal. It's time to knock iron off this pedestal. Our faith in iron as an energizer, a strengthener, has been misplaced.

It's impossible to say how many early American colonists and pioneers may have been affected by cooking in iron skillets and drinking high iron well water. On the other hand, pioneers were not threatened on every side by excessive iron added to their breakfast cereals and other foods. Cereal killers. The pioneer families of the little houses on the prairies didn't face the menace of sitting down every morning to a breakfast cereal that boasted, "one hundred percent of your day's requirement."

It is not hard to get enough iron. It may be more difficult not to get too much. To keep from storing too much iron from your food, your metabolism for iron has to be near perfect. Unfortunately, a slight defect can cause you to absorb a little more than you need day by day.

Crosby says, "The ability to absorb only what the body needs is to have a normal iron metabolism."

The RDA (recommended daily allowance) or RDI (recommended daily intake) is a matter we'll take up later.

How would you like to win the genetic lottery? In my view the H gene is the best of abnormal genes to carry. Since you'll know exactly what to do. Just be sure to do it!

Victor Herbert led the Nutrition Symposium at the 1987 meeting of the American College of Physicians. "It's not what we don't know about nutrition that hurts us," he said. "It's what we know for sure that's dead wrong."

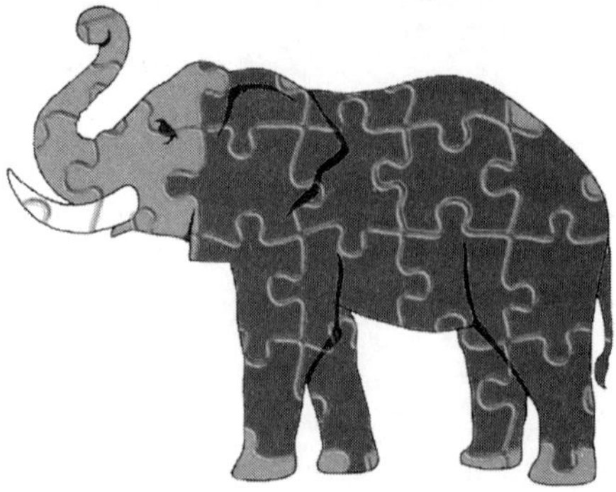

Part 5

"How would I find out if I have it?"

Chapter 15

The Eight Hurdles

The million and a half Americans included in twenty-five million of the world's people, who unknowingly are accumulating deadly iron stores face eight hurdles to the early detection and adequate treatment that could save them. The lucky few who clear all eight hurdles will avoid organ destruction from iron damage and live out a normal life span, barring other misfortunes. In most cases their good luck will be at the expense of relatives who were not so fortunate, the Sacrificial Siblings.

The typical undiagnosed iron loading person is entirely unaware that he is smashing into hurdle after hurdle. He may vaguely recognize that something is wrong, but he never heard of hemochromatosis.

Hurdle Number One: Iron levels not tested.

*Paul, a young Connecticut man, employed by a prestigious oil company, received medical care as part of his employment benefits. His annual physical examination was thorough, it was "complete," but it did *not* include the simple blood tests for iron that would have indicated abnormal levels. Paul was not diagnosed and treated, and as a result, became disabled at 42.

The tests that Paul was given should have included serum iron (SI) together with Total Iron Binding Capacity (TIBC). The lab should then have divided the TIBC into the SI to arrive at the percentage of transferrin saturation. It's the proportion of these two numbers that is significant. You're looking for a normal range of 12 to 45 percent. If the lab does not make this computation, the physician should. If he doesn't, the patient must.

These measurements are taken from blood samples that are tested in the blood chemistry profiles.

Another blood test that is being used increasingly is called the UIBC, unsaturated iron binding capacity. It can be used as an initial test. UIBC is readily automated, the reagent costs pennies and reliability is good. You calculate the TIBC by adding UIBC to serum iron.

UIBC can identify both excessive and low levels of iron. Jerome L. Sullivan, MD, PhD, says he likes the UIBC. It's easier to automate, and it does a great job of detecting low levels. Low levels would be seen in cases of high transferrin saturation. So hemochromatosis patients generally have low UIBC. Sullivan would like to see blood banks "do a UIBC on every volunteer blood donor and write the result on the blood bag for clinicians to see." He said, "This would serve both as a screen of the donor population for hemochromatosis and as a guide to clinicians who want to transfuse plasma that is rich in UIBC to certain patients."

Sullivan said UIBC is potentially easier to understand, the higher the number the better. The higher the UIBC the greater the chance that the patient is genetically normal. He said that transferrin saturation requires "inverse thinking." Increased levels are worse. With UIBC you are talking about a positive something, i.e. free transferrin. "With transferrin saturation, a number that speaks to the relationship between iron and transferrin," Sullivan said, "there needs to be additional mental processing by the patient/doctor to work out its meaning." He added, "The disadvantage of UIBC is that it is unfamiliar to most physicians and most laboratories. There would need to be a very significant educational effort to establish its widespread use."

Dr. Virgil F. Fairbanks of Mayo Clinic is strongly critical of examinations that don't even include serum iron. "... it is ridiculous," he says, "that we measure serum sodium and potassium routinely in ambulatory patients when we should be measuring serum iron concentration instead."

Paul filed a lawsuit against his employer and has since received a settlement of one and a half million dollars.

*A Marco Island, Florida man had received two hip replacements in 1971. He also suffered many of the other problems that should have made somebody think of iron, but no iron tests were given, not until 1984, when it was belatedly discovered that the patient's problem was too much iron.

*Mark, a thirty-year-old South Dakota man, had suffered a virus that he couldn't overcome. It was diagnosed as mononucleosis. After the sore throat and fever left, he continued to have trouble with headache, bowels and "complete fatigue." His skin was hot to the touch. It broke out in red splotches. Pains appeared off and on in his side. Then he noticed some instances of memory failure.

His doctors were at a loss. Mark said he had to fight with four doctors; he had to travel a thousand miles before he finally received a diagnosis. Physicians had failed to test iron levels.

*A Trenton, New Jersey man, 51, was diagnosed, "just by luck" after he had sought help from two orthopedists, two neurologists, three neurosurgeons, three therapists. A slipped disc had started his downward spiral, but, although he was told he had "the back of an eighty-year-old," no one tested him for iron. Finally a physician was suspicious of his dark skin color and the enlarged liver.

*In East Point, Georgia, "My husband had always complained of this and that hurting," wrote Mrs. C. "It was always something different: stomach, back, eyes, head. He had several physicals, but nothing was ever found to treat."

Even after he developed diabetes, his iron was not checked. Finally, *finally* — after a liver biopsy, the iron tests were made. By then his serum ferritin was 4,783. Normal range is to 150. Vigorous treatment began, and "We thank God for my husband's excellent health today," his wife says. But she adds, "We feel he would have been spared a great deal of pain and illness ... if the doctors had found his problem years sooner." The patient's two brothers and son all benefitted by receiving early diagnoses.

The blood tests for iron are not perfect. Iron levels do fluctuate from day to day and from hour to hour. This simple first step, however, is saving lives. When transferrin saturation persists above 45 percent, a test for serum ferritin should be ordered. Serum ferritin levels above 150 should lead to further investigation.

Had Paul received proper blood tests for iron in his annual company physical he would have cleared Hurdle Number One and possibly he would not have suffered the sad outcome of being totally disabled by age forty-two. The company physicians would have been spared an expensive lawsuit.

Better yet, we can remove that first hurdle entirely. Let's include transferrin saturation or UIBC in all routine physicals. Not cost effective? Ask any belatedly diagnosed patient if it would have been cost effective. Ask a patient who was diagnosed early, who is healthy and well if the test was cost effective.

One major laboratory began including iron panels in its routine Chemscreen in 1990. MetPath Laboratories, now Quest, with headquarters in New Jersey, are now instrumental in the life-saving diagnosis of thousands of people. Within the first few months half a million tests revealed one in a hundred iron abnormalities.

In most medical offices the iron iceberg lurks unseen.

*Rhonda in Hot Springs Arkansas is right to worry about her son who requires transfusions, which she knows will pack him with dangerous amounts of iron, and unknowing physicians are giving him ferrous sulfate at the rate of 972 milligrams daily.

*A physician in Miami told Arlene to give her husband Ensure. "It's loaded with iron," he said, "which couldn't hurt." Eight years and eleven doctors later, Phil was diagnosed.

*From Blacklick Ohio: "I went to two doctors asking to have my iron tested, and they both laughed and said there is no such disease."

*Joann in Salinas California took her mother to a doctor and gave him information from IOD. He shrugged. Two years later she went elsewhere and was diagnosed and was then awaiting a liver transplant.

Laughs and shrugs. We hear about both frequently.

On Sept 19, 1993 *60 MINUTES* aired a show that put our cause back half a decade. They did not realize they were doing that. In fact, their research was so shallow it made me see television in a new light, even though I had worked in TV a number of years. Advertisers have all the power in TV, unlike newspapers, which do try to maintain distance between their sales and editorials staffs.

60 MINUTES rightly likes to point out scams and wastes of money. In this case they pointed the finger at medical labs that do too much testing, especially those that test ferritin. Lesley Stahl on closeup asked, "What is ferritin anyway?"

IOD members across the country who knew that their accidental diagnosis came only because their ferritin was measured, were outraged. They flooded *60 MINUTES* with letters of protest. We had for years tried to interest the program into doing a program. In order for that to happen one of three things would have had to take place. One of the decision makers would have had bitter knowledge himself because of losing a family member .. Or .. There would have been some way to help a sponsor make more money (sell less iron?) .. Or someone on the staff would have had to have enough imagination to understand this as a serious and urgent problem. It is really surprising how little imagination you find in the media.

We invited *60 MINUTES* to visit our offices to answer our phones and read our mail. We told them it would open their eyes and break their hearts.

From Rye New Hampshire Elizabeth wrote that her husband died in 1989, diagnosed one week before death. He had seen an internist for 30 years for high blood pressure. Cancer developed in pancreas, liver, spine, and lungs. An oncologist told the family not to worry about their daughter because women are not affected, only men.

After reading an Ann Landers column from IOD the women decided to be tested. Three sisters were then diagnosed. That cheered IOD, but at the same time we sagged, remembering the nine years of day and night work before their brother died. Elizabeth said, "I only wish we knew about IOD before my husband was so badly damaged." We sadly said that getting media attention is like chipping through granite.

Media exposure can do wonders. IOD member Bob Joyce was riding in an elevator in the Cook County Building in Chicago one day in March 1996. He heard a conversation between two men.

"My son has been quite ill for some time. He's had many complaints and has seen numerous doctors, but none of the doctors could diagnose what was wrong." The man continued in a worried voice, "During all this time my son was becoming sicker and sicker." He turned and tapped his companion gleefully. "Well, guess what? I was watching CBS late news one night and I saw an interview with a Chicagoan named Jack Connor. He was on the air with Dr Warren Fury - it was on the Dr Michael Breen Show. Watching this show it occurred to me that my son had many of the symptoms these people were describing.

"So I took my son to a doctor and requested the tests that were named." He nodded with satisfaction. "That was it! My son had something called hemochromatosis. The best part is there's an easy treatment. My son is now starting aggressive treatment - and I feel sure he's going to be all right!"

Mrs W of Nedrow New York expressed much sympathy when she heard about the death of Tom Walsh at age 37. "It should be mandatory," she said, "for doctors to test for iron."

We heard from a physician in Mercer Island Washington. R. E. Buckingham Jr MD said, "I am stupefied that there is no much ignorance in the medical and lay community over a common treatable condition which, left untreated, can lead to serious problems, even death."

David L Witte MD PhD made a presentation in 1990 at a seminar for College of American Pathology in Dallas. He said that "few life-threatening diseases ... have such an innocuous, inexpensive and effective therapy." He said, "Since removal of iron by phlebotomy can stop the disease's advance and even restore organ health, the patient, pathologist and physician can all rejoice." Witte admitted that labs may find more "false positives than true positives," but he added, "All the true positives will help an entire kindred forever."

Hurdle Number Two: Iron tests given but not properly interpreted.

Serum iron assay is beginning to appear more often in chemistry profiles, but that test by itself is not informative enough. It needs the TIBC to reveal transferrin saturation. However, serum iron is better than nothing, and an SI value above 145 must be followed up. Tests are useless of course if they are ignored.

"I never heard of this disease until I was told I had it," writes Mrs. H of Dallas, Texas. Her iron levels were tested during a physical, and tests revealed a serum ferritin of 885. Mrs. H was advised to avoid red meats and substitute cheese dishes. A later ferritin tested at 567 and a subsequent test showed 771. "But the doctor told me not to worry about it," she said.

*Amy was tested at a Florida health fair. Luckily the tests included serum iron. Hurdle Number One cleared. Amy's test results were normal except for high SI. The lab comment was: serum iron abnormally high, could indicate disease. See your physician.

Unluckily for Amy she crashed into Hurdle Number Two when her doctor said, "I'd rather have high iron than low." Airily waving away a test result leaves a patient wondering why a test is done if the result is going to be disregarded. That doctor visit left Amy uneasy, but she didn't have enough information about iron to protect herself.

The misconception that high iron levels are healthier than low iron is still prevalent in the medical profession. The patient's only protection is to understand the true role of iron in the human body. The patient must insist on iron tests. Then the patient must not ignore abnormal levels.

*Madeline in Leesburg Florida was misdiagnosed for years. She tested with high iron and even high liver enzymes, but the numbers were ignored. She was put on tranquilizers. She was sent to a psychiatrist. Then at 40, after developing diabetes, she finally got a diagnosis.

*Lee was told by a number of physicians that he was a hypochondriac. Finally he demanded, "Do a battery of tests and find out what's wrong!" So the tests were done and they did include iron.

"Here are your results," said the doctor, "perfectly normal." He tossed the lab report across the desk. Lee examined the report. "This 1200 ferritin," he said, "is that normal?" Another diagnosis finally made because the patient persisted. Lee wrote IOD, "Why do doctors order lab tests and then ignore the results?"

*Mary of Santa Rosa California says that her three hip surgeries and severe arthritis could have been prevented if her physician had "carefully read the lab report eight years prior."

Hurdle Number Three: The anemic iron overloaded patient may be given additional iron.

I grew up in Indiana, where I enjoyed a healthy childhood, with one exception. I was anemic, pale, underweight, easily tired. Anemia is determined by the number, color, size, shape and life span of red blood cells, hemoglobin levels and percentage of hematocrit. Doctors saw the anemic child and prescribed iron. They *assumed* "iron deficiency anemia."

When I started working in radio and television and I was moving about, I saw physicians in other states. Doctors continued the iron therapy, and when the "run down" condition worsened instead of improving, doctors *increased* the iron (Trinsicon). Some of the vitamins in the Trinsicon did bring about some temporary improvement. Meanwhile the iron's insidious destruction remained hidden. Clinicians criticize that kind of therapy. They say it clouds the whole picture and makes it almost impossible to assess results. I did and do respond to folic acid and vitamin B12. As it turns out, deficiencies of folic acid and B12 or B6 are specific iron-loading anemias.

It was the excess iron that was causing the pallor, weight loss and fatigue.

*Pat in Lakeside, California, was an anemic child who was given Tastyeast and various "things to build me up." In the early 1940s the company doctor where she worked gave her liver shots for the anemia and she took iron tablets. One of her early symptoms was diarrhea off and on for three years until it became uncontrollable.

Pat also began suffering episodes of weakness and nervousness that go along with hypoglycemia. Claus Niederau, MD, PhD, once reported at an IOD symposium that this low blood sugar is often present in the pre-cirrhotic stage and accompanies hyperinsulism. The pancreas responds to stimulus such as sugar or caffeine by putting out too much insulin, which in turn causes a sharp drop in the blood sugar level.

Many patients have told IOD of these periods of low blood sugar, although very little is mentioned in the medical literature.

Pat is one of many hemochromatosis patients who suffered mild anemia of unidentified origin — not the severe iron loading anemias. These patients were medicated with iron.

IOD's 1988 survey revealed that twenty-four percent of diagnosed hemochromatosis patients were anemic. Doctors had medicated them with iron!

"I am seventy-four-years-old," writes Beth from Tucson, Arizona, "and for quite some time my doctor has been giving me iron medicine because I am anemic. Now he tells me that my system has too much iron, and I have regularly to have blood drained from me ..."

From Buffalo, New York, "In 1972 I first went to ... a highly regarded rheumatologist ... with pain in my hands and left ankle and foot. He diagnosed my condition as rheumatoid arthritis and began treating me with anti-inflammatory steroids. I did not tolerate steroids well because of a previous history of GI ulcers. So he began a series of colloidal gold injections which were continued through 1977.

"Early in the course of this therapy, (the doctor) found that I was chronically anemic with a persistent low hematocrit. He prescribed an iron supplement which I then took daily for about five years. I am not aware that he ever had any blood work done to measure iron levels ... In 1977 my foot became so painful that I was referred to an orthopedic surgeon ... who recommended that my ankle be fused. Before submitting to this I sought a second opinion ... and saw another orthopedic surgeon. At the time ... the doctor examined my foot and ankle, and he commented about my facial complexion which he described as coppery, and asked if I would see an internist colleague ... I was seen by the internist ... and a rheumatologist ... They obtained extensive blood tests and brought another doctor for consultation, a hematologist ... It was then I first heard of hemochromatosis ...

"The most distressing aspect of all this is that (the first rheumatologist) not only failed to correctly diagnose my condition but the iron supplements which he prescribed during the five-six years he treated me undoubtedly contributed to the severity of the iron load in my body." She noted that a fraternal twin sister has also been diagnosed, but that her complications are much milder.

While serving in the military, George was medicated with Feosol for a "mild anemia." That was during the late 1940s. Later in Japan George experienced debilitating liver trouble. Doctors were somewhat confused, but called it hepatitis. By age fifty-two diabetes developed. When George happened to be hospitalized for a viral infection, an internist took a personal interest. He said, "Why should an underweight man of fifty-two require so much insulin?" A liver biopsy revealed the answer. Hemochromatosis!

During treatment severe arthritis entered the picture. Most of George's doctors had not bothered with testing Total Iron Binding Capacity (TIBC), but had been content with serum iron assays. Worse, "...most of my doctors have tended to fear phlebotomies," George says.

Elyane, a patient in Austin, Texas, received a visit from her sister in France. "French doctors had been giving her iron supplements..." While she was in Austin she was suffering various complaints and her sister took her to an Austin physician who made the correct diagnosis of hemochromatosis. But it was too late. She died five years later. How or whether she was treated after her return to France is not known. Her sister's diagnosis then led to Elyane's.

*Josephine in Dunedin Florida was prescribed iron for 20 years for anemia. After one day testing with a ferritin of 1236 she was told to try an iron free diet. Her doctor in confusion told her, "You can't have high iron when you're anemic."

Confusion is epidemic. A blood bank in Stockton California told Aurora she has too much iron. How high? They said 17.6.

Blood banks don't measure iron. They measure hemoglobin or hematocrit. But they don't know the difference.

Dietitians and nutritionists continue to publish newspaper columns telling the public how to get more iron in the diet. An overwhelming ignorance persists. Very few seem to realize that any ordinary diet is loaded with excess iron. They fail to realize the importance of metabolism. A normal metabolism for iron can exercise its ability to *refrain* from absorbing excess. They don't understand that many people lack this ability. They don't even know that iron is not excreted.

The most ignored fact of all is that a number of anemias are iron loading.

Sylvia Bottomley MD, Professor of Medicine at University of Oklahoma describes the condition as an abnormality in the bone marrow in which iron is not properly used to form heme in the red cell. So the mineral accumulates in a section of the cell that damages the red cell. Many of these cells never make it into the blood stream. Hence the anemia.

The iron has to go somewhere. Since iron can't be excreted, it must be stored.

Bottomley advises patients to in some cases improve the anemia with vitamin B6 (pyridoxine). She warns that the excess iron must be treated, removed. "In persons with mild anemia the iron excess is easily removed with appropriately scheduled and supervised phlebotomies despite the anemia," she says. More severely anemic patients who require regular transfusions must be treated with desferrioxamine (Desferal) to chelate the iron. Chelation is not the treatment of choice. However it's all that's available to those who have severe anemia.

Hurdle Number Four: Failure to stain liver biopsy specimen to reveal iron.

Walter G. Frey, III, MD, presented a detailed method for determining a quantitative measurement of liver iron by needle biopsy in the Journal of Laboratory and Clinical Medicine (Vol. 72, No. 1, 52-57, July 1968).

Before that time quantitative studies had not been usual, but Frey said such studies could prove of value in studying the progression of iron storage diseases and in evaluating the efficacy of therapy. Frey criticized earlier methods of determining the amount of liver iron in necropsy specimens as inaccurate. Of course by the time of necropsy the patient is dead. However, the family needs the information. Sometimes the liver specimen is not properly stained, and the iron is missed altogether.

IOD no longer says that it is essential to undergo liver biopsy. We stopped recommending it as necessary after too many stories poured in with a variety of difficulties. Many do go very well. I had two biopsies with no problem whatsoever. But IOD hears from more patients hourly and worldwide than anyone else. We also know of a study that says one in 1,000 people die from just this medical procedure. Weigh that loss against any possible gain. When a physician does take a tiny sample of your liver he may tell you that, yes, you do have cirrhosis. He will not suggest any treatment. There is none that I have heard of except to get rid of the iron as fast as possible. You need to do that anyway, once you discover the iron.

Virgil Fairbanks, MD, of the Mayo Clinic says, "When a patient, informed of the risk, declines a liver biopsy, the physician must so note in the record and then treat on the assumption of hemochromatosis."

James of Lincoln City, Oregon, said that after a doctor asks you to sign the form regarding the risk, James might say to him, "I need to inform you up front that there is a known three percent possibility of generating a malpractice complication with this procedure."

A physician on the Internet wrote, "I also do not believe that a liver biopsy is always necessary. .... Since I rationalized that I would need phlebotomies regardless of my liver iron stores, it made no sense because my treatment would not be affected by the biopsy results..."

Charley of Madison, New Jersey, suffered a frozen shoulder three days following his liver biopsy.

Laura Sullivan MD of Winter Park, Florida, wrote, "Liver biopsy should not be required for diagnosis, because some patients may refuse the biopsy and delay much needed treatment."

Another from the Internet: "...(my grandfather) died from complications during the procedure when the doctor knicked a bile duct with the needle." Several other members of the family were then diagnosed, but declined the biopsy.

Other stories that came to us include various body parts punctured; the biopsy failing to show the iron and the diagnosis missed and a number of deaths. We can't help feeling that the benefit of the liver biopsy is not worth the problems, not to mention the unnecessary expense.

Corwin Edwards at IOD's 16th Annual Symposium listed reasons that make the liver biopsy no longer the gold standard for diagnosis. He said biopsies on advanced cases missed eight percent of the diagnosis, and worse, that half of the biopsies were normal on early pre-symptomatic cases.

A Florida neurologist underwent a liver biopsy to rule out cancer, after tests showed abnormal liver enzyme levels. "Good news," his beaming gastroenterologist reported. "No cancer." Luckily, a physician friend was in town visiting. He asked to take a look at the specimen. "Mmmmh ... what's all that sandy stuff ..." Could it be iron? A Prussian blue stain was applied to reveal liver iron. Because of his friend's visit, the neurologist lived for another thirty years. Hemochromatosis was well known by a few doctors as long ago as the 1940s.

The patient, himself a doctor, cleared Hurdle Number Four by the skin of his liver because someone wondered: could it be iron. If they don't suspect it, they don't look for it ...

Vincent Felitti MD is screening and treating thousands at Kaiser Permanente in San Diego. He said, "I cannot think of a case where a liver biopsy would have helped."

Hurdle Number Five: The symptoms aren't right.

A Chicago corporation executive gave up his career when he became disabled as a result of delayed diagnosis. After years of misdiagnosis, he found a doctor who helped him leap over Hurdles One, Two, Three, and Four. But the doctor erected in his path Hurdle Number Five.

Mike's test results showed high iron and were correctly interpreted. Mike was not anemic; he was not given iron. The liver biopsy was stained and iron was found in abundance.

At this point most people would have received a correct diagnosis. However, Mike's doctor took from his shelf a medical text and looked up "hemochromatosis." He shook his head. "I thought you had this rare disease," he said. "But for that you need diabetes. No, it isn't hemochromatosis." (That dirty fifteen letter word!)

Medical texts are filled with such dusty information about "classic triads: diabetes, skin pigmentation and enlarged (liver, heart)." New writers continue to quote misinformation, and the dangerous myths live on.

Mike was left entangled in Hurdle Number Five until he was later rescued with a diagnosis, which, however, was too late to restore him to health and career.

William H. Crosby, MD, reminds us that "Hemochromatosis does occur without any of these complications..." He says, "One most serious misconception is that a diagnosis of hemochromatosis can be made only when the disease is fully developed, ie, when the accumulation of iron has caused damage to the storage organs."

Hurdle Number Six: Timid treatment.

You sail over the five hurdles and receive a proper diagnosis only to trip over Hurdle Number Six. There are doctors who can't bring themselves to take your money and your blood! Yet detection is only part of your battle, and diagnosis alone will not save your life.

IOD offices receive many reports from patients whose doctors are giving Timid Treatment. The patient needs to unload the iron as fast as possible. Phlebotomies should be scheduled weekly, twice weekly or even oftener if tolerated. This kind of therapy requires some adjustment on the part of the patient, and he'll snatch at any excuse to postpone the bloodletting. Heart trouble, fatigue, pain. The patient must remind himself where all this distress is coming from.

Doctors and the family should reinforce the patient's motivation. The actual treatment is similar to making a donation at the blood bank. When you first hear a description of the treatment, you are jolted by a shock. But it turns out to be less dire than it sounds.

Correct treatment will be discussed in more detail later.

Physicians are giving patients much misinformation. Richard

of Sarasota Florida was told he brought on his hemochromatosis by drinking alcohol. He doesn't drink.

Hurdle Number Seven: Disbelief.

Bernice of Pineville, North Carolina, was properly tested following the diagnosis of her sister, who had received a "stringent examination" on her entrance into a retirement facility. Bernice's tests did show high iron and a liver/spleen scan was also abnormal. Still she hesitated to agree to a liver biopsy because "I have not up to this time shown any symptoms."

It is understandable that the patient may sometimes doubt that he has a disease that no one ever heard of. A sense of unreality falls around you. In the first months of IOD's organizing, I was struck by moments of doubt. How could I, a layman, discover facts about a disorder so unknown by medical professionals? We were at that time hearing constant reports of doctors waving off their patients' request for tests with, "I never heard of it."

As a journalist, I had a horror of losing my way down a thorny pathway toward facts that might prove to be mirages. Yet as we caught up with those facts, they turned out to be standing on solid foundations. Scientific studies from the labs continued to fortify the findings. And the letters and calls from belatedly diagnosed patients kept coming in a stream that sometimes became a flood.

The patient is in shock after being told he has this unheard of disease. He's the first in the family to be discovered. He is especially vulnerable to doubt if his diagnosis has been made before organ damage. "How can I have a fatal disease if I feel all right?" he argues. He can often find a doctor to share his disbelief. Old criteria for a diagnosis do require cirrhosis, heart or pancreas damage, or skin pigmentation.

If the patient begins searching, he'll have no trouble locating a doctor who will reassure him. "I don't believe you have hemochromatosis. Let's make some more tests and wait six months to see what happens."

It happened to Susanna. Her husband divorced her because of her hemochromatosis. Treatment had cured the diabetes, however she lost her insurance and became indigent. Her new physician told her she does not have that awful H word. He refused to treat for two years. The diabetes returned. Many who take the DNA test get kicked out of treatment because the genes that turn up don't satisfy the physician. In Susanna's case, though, she did have the expected genes and the doctor was forced to admit that yes, indeed, she does have the disease. Treatment has resumed, and Susanna can only hope that her diabetes will again go away.

When enough time goes by and enough irreversible injury has occurred, both patient and doctor may be satisfied to say, "Now it's hemochromatosis."

Rodney in Florida was told he does not really have hemochromatosis. This after a confirming liver biopsy plus three months of weekly phlebotomies plus diagnosis of relatives. What more does that doctor want?

Hurdle Number Eight: Failure to check relatives.

Rose's brother had died of hemochromatosis. Rose suffered several symptoms that kept worsening: arthritis, gastric problems, fatigue. She pointed out to doctors that her brother's symptoms were similar. Shouldn't she be tested? No, no, it's not a woman's disease. The myths simply won't die!

Rose became more and more alarmed. She contacted IOD for counseling. Should she go to a famous clinic, she wondered. She lived in North Dakota. A good idea, she was advised, but the individual physician, not the institution, makes the difference between correct and incorrect diagnosis of iron overload.

The iron-aware physician whom Rose consulted made a prompt diagnosis of hemochromatosis. Rose had strung along with her previous physicians for eight years! Her brother had been the Sacrificial Sibling, but his sacrifice had almost proved futile. Every "complete" physical should include iron tests, properly interpreted. In the presence of symptoms, iron should always be suspected and ruled out. Relatives *must* be monitored.

A Palm Beach man used to worry about iron overload when it cost the life of his brother. But Ken got little satisfaction from his doctor, who told him, "Stop worrying." His iron was tested, serum iron only. It was high, sometimes 171 or 255. Ken decided to accept his physician's advice. He stopped worrying. A few years later, however, after his physician retired, his new doctor made the diagnosis.

Mr. R, now in Brazil, wrote that the persistence of an outstanding person, a Philadelphia physician, "lead to my discovery, subsequent treatment and my good health today." The doctor had pursued investigation of the entire family after a combination of sideroblastic anemia and hemochromatosis was found in a family member.

Ethel in California was another lucky patient who received an early diagnosis as a result of family screening. At the time of her diagnosis, she says, "I was in perfect health, at best weight ever ..." Still she feels that a subsequent gall bladder removal and a mastectomy are related to hemochromatosis. What would have been the case with an even earlier diagnosis...?

James in Winter Park, Florida, has diabetes. A liver biopsy revealed a "dark spot" that doctors said was iron. James' younger brother also has diabetes. Another brother has been diagnosed with hemochromatosis. James' doctor told him not to worry because his "body functions would eliminate the iron." Patients' relatives must receive vigorous investigation. In the absence of symptoms and with blood tests that show normal levels, the relatives nevertheless can sometimes be diagnosed after persistent checking.

Margaret in St Augustine Florida persisted with 25 physicians before she could receive a correct diagnosis.

Courtney of Memphis had lost her brother to this condition. He was diagnosed but was told there was no treatment. When Courtney began experiencing some of the same symptoms she visited her brother's physician. He sadly told her she did indeed have the disease and she would be dead in two years. Courtney had already seen what the condition could do, so she believed the doctor. She settled all her affairs and gave away everything. She gave all her money to her mother. Then she found IOD. We told her she would not die, but instead would be intensively treated. Since then Courtney has remarried and has survived.

Relatives of diagnosed patients are not always content with blood tests that show "normal" iron levels. Walter Frey has ordered liver biopsies on relatives that confirmed the diagnosis, after blood tests were normal.

There is no substitute for a correct diagnosis. The alternative is unacceptable. Sickness and death.

IOD had been chipping away at a granite mountain of ignorance and misconceptions for ten years when a 29-year-old Jacksonville Florida woman died and was diagnosed at autopsy. Despite our work we lacked the resources to reach everybody.

We did not ask the public to help us find a cure. We had one. An easy one. All that was needed was awareness. We asked many celebrities to join our effort. We happened to know of several who had been lucky enough to be diagnosed and were being treated. Not one of them was willing to share that good luck with other people. I think I will never be able to understand that.

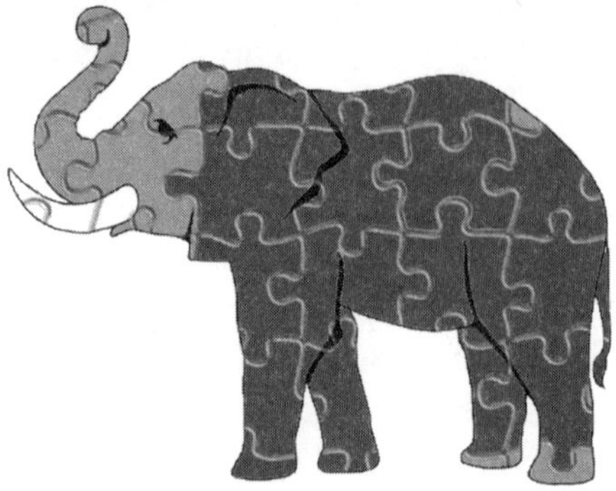

Chapter 16

The Trouble With Symptoms

One of the first questions you'll ask about a disease is, "What are the symptoms?" In fact, quite often in the early stages there are *no* symptoms.

Discussing the list of symptoms associated with hemochromatosis is as risky as the word itself, and for the same reason. The practitioner who requires a set of symptoms to fit the word is likely to misdiagnose an iron overloaded patient whose symptoms vary from the preconceived "full-blown case."

Because of the wide-ranging damage, symptoms can be many. They can come and go. "My side aches, my back, my hands ..." The next visit, "severe headaches," and the one after that, "too tired to drag around," then "my sex life is shot," or "diarrhea."

The diagnostician makes plenty of tests, he treats the symptoms, but he misses the diagnosis, unless he suspects iron.

The weary patient who consults a physician because of fatigue is in a communication bind. Who isn't tired? The overworked doctor may be thinking, "Tell me about it!" The patient himself does not realize the extent of his tiredness, that it is a desperate kind of fatigue that you can't rest away. He probably suffers guilt at being unable to overcome the lethargy the way other people do. *They're* tired, too. He hears it every day, "I'm dead." Yet those people don't cave in. Why can't I snap out of it? worries the patient. Wouldn't it make sense for sufferers of "chronic fatigue syndrome" to get their iron tested?

Liver malfunction and inability to metabolize protein can lead to problems of memory and concentration. Skin pigmentation can occur: coloration can be bronze or take on a dull grayish cast.

Walter Frey remarked at a Florida meeting that he had seen more "bronze" skins of patients that day than in his years of practice in New Hampshire. "In our part of the country," he said, "the color is more often an ashy gray." He remembered that one patient had been called by the nickname, Whitey, because of his grayish appearance.

Patients send to IOD information that is not mentioned in the medical literature. Dark skin color has been reported on the face at the inside corners of eyes and creases at outer nostrils. The literature says pigmentation appears on exposed areas, and places of indentations, such as underarms, inside elbows, backs of hands, rectum and perineal area. Patients say darkening appears in "places where the sun don't shine."

The maze of symptoms are so nonspecific and baffling that often the patient is dismissed with a prescription for tranquilizers. One Texas physician saw a patient (undiagnosed hemochromatosis patient) in his waiting room, and sighed, "Is she here again?" The patient overheard the remark and decided to give up going to doctors. She died some time later in the hospital, where her diagnosis was finally made.

What if there are no symptoms? The liver is a heroic organ. It struggles on despite everything that's thrown at it. Even after injury, the liver strives to repair itself. By the time the enlargement is noticed, there is considerable damage. Liver function tests reflect abnormalities long after the beginning of the injury.

The best time to receive a diagnosis of hemochromatosis is before any symptoms. If you find you have excess iron, but no symptoms, fine. Unload the iron and enjoy your good health.

There have been instances of patients whose liver contained enough iron that they rang alarms at airport security checkpoints. If those detectors were only more sensitive to catch early cases — if only the detectors were standardized. Well, maybe the SQUID will be the answer. The superconducting quantum-interference device measures iron through the magnetic field produced by the human body. The SQUID is one of the diagnostic tools being developed by high tech research.

Occasionally patients are diagnosed through magnetic resonance imaging, formerly called nuclear magnetic resonance. The MRI can show density of the liver. With the right equipment and the right technicians, a diagnosis is possible. A few patients have been detected by CAT scans.

Incontrovertible proof of excess iron is simply: can you have withdrawn a pint of blood weekly for four to six weeks and not become persistently anemic during this time? If so, you are iron overloaded. What is the indicator of anemia? For adult women it is hemoglobin less than 12 or hematocrit less than 36 percent. For men normal hemoglobin ranges from 12 to 16; hematocrit, 40 to 45 percent.

There is plenty of disagreement about various aspects of iron overload among the authorities. Some of their views are presented in these pages for your consideration. Let's try to put together the pieces of this iron elephant. Everybody still has much to learn.

Crosby, speaking at our Tenth Annual Symposium, held in West Palm Beach, explained that about the time of the Civil War a case of hemochromatosis was discovered at autopsy. The patient had cirrhosis. Hemochromatosis was described as a disease of cirrhosis, bronze diabetes and pigmented skin. They were still saying that as late as 1875, "and that description has stuck," said Dr. Crosby. "Give me a break!"

A woman in Louisiana had lost her brother from this condition. She herself suffered diabetes and "twelve times the normal amount of iron in the liver." In frustration she cried, "but I don't have cirrhosis yet and my doctor said the definition of hemochromatosis is excess iron with cellular damage."

Donna in Cheswick Pennsylvania is now on crutches because her HLA did not fit her physician's faulty perception. Donna's A2 and B27 is one we hear about all the time. But the medical literature is over focused on A3 and B7 or B14. Donna's brother died at age 35 of liver problems. When Donna's ferritin reached 750 her doctor shook his head. He wanted to see more than 1,000. Well, he did. His comment: "I don't know where all this iron is coming from." Donna now has vascular necrosis, has had bone transplant and expense exceeding $17,000. She says her insurance company is also a victim. It covered her all the years while she was undiagnosed.

The entire insurance industry is part of the problem. Its ignorance is as deep as the medical community's. The word hemochromatosis sets a flag on a client. They cancel the policy and if they don't cancel they refuse to cover phlebotomy. I tell them they are reckless and foolish and throwing money away. **Most patients are undiagnosed.** As in Donna's case they are covering undiagnosed people and spending unnecessary money.

Marylyn in San Jose says she now knows why "the men in the family died before age 60." Since her brother's death, diagnoses have been made on herself, her 32-year-old daughter, her 29-year-old son and their first cousin.

In 1995 a big controversy developed regarding the necessity for a liver biopsy. Guess who decided the biopsy is required and refuse to treat without "establishing a diagnosis:" the liver specialists and gastroenterologists, those who actually performed the procedure. Most others had gradually come around to the fact that it was not only not essential, but that there were several reasons to skip it, since the risk to life was about one in a thousand. Other complications could develop. It could even miss the diagnosis.

Jerome Sullivan wrote, "A liver biopsy should not be required for hemochromatosis patients before starting treatment. If stored iron were essential for life and its removal were dangerous, it might make sense to make the patient and his doctor jump through one more hoop before starting a course of phlebotomy. But *stored* iron is not essential for life and its removal may lower the risk of heart attack, cancer, and some serious infectious diseases, even in people who do not have hemochromatosis by strict criteria.

"If a patient does not truly have hemochromatosis, this will become clear early during a course of phlebotomies. All that will be lost is a lot of excess stored iron that is not needed and may be harmful. What iron overloaded patients do not need are overly narrow and restrictive criteria for the diagnosis.

"The safety of liver biopsy is not the main issue, although, clearly, removing blood from a vein is much safer than inserting a large bore needle into the liver. In the real world, insistence on a liver biopsy may delay diagnosis and treatment. Many patients are reluctant to do it. The doctor who refuses to treat without the biopsy may discourage the patient from pursuing the matter, especially if he/she is not yet symptomatic. That delay may mean delay too for affected relatives."

Sullivan wrote, "Demanding a costly liver biopsy puts one more block in the road to timely diagnosis and treatment."

The controversy continued to rage.

At IOD's 14th Annual Symposium held in St Louis, a debate was presented between Bruce Bacon MD and Sullivan.

Dr Bacon maintained that "you need the biopsy to distinguish between homozygotes and heterozygotes." He presented four cases where ferritin and saturation were elevated, but where the biopsy revealed no iron stain on the liver.

Sullivan said the biopsy may sometimes be necessary, but should not be a "knee jerk decision." He pointed out that missing the diagnosis of an incurable disease does little harm, but delay the diagnosis of a disease that is "curable" if caught early? Big mistake. He said the biopsy can miss the iron, and the consequences of a false negative means the disease progresses. The patient dies. The family is not alerted. He added, "Refusal to treat patients who refuse the biopsy is unacceptable."

Kathleen in Cocoa Beach, Florida, had no insurance and could not afford the liver biopsy. Her doctor dismissed her, saying he could not begin treatment without a diagnosis. As her symptoms worsened she actually felt she was dying. Finally another physician made the diagnosis and started treatment. Later much improved and engaged to be married, Kathleen said, "I never thought I would live this long."She is now well, married and happy.

In March 1997 the Centers for Disease Control (CDC) held a meeting in Atlanta. Ernest Beutler MD said, "If I asked those who think a liver biopsy is essential to move to the right side of the room, and those who believe a phlebotomy program is adequate to move to the left, I suspect that most hematologists and other doctors would be on the left – and gastroenterologists on the right." He paused. "The risk is not low."

An unexpected symptom of excess iron is anemia. Iron loading anemias are much more common than is recognized. The myth that iron deficiency is the "world's most common nutritional problem" has a strangle hold on the medical community, even World Health Organization (WHO).

But let's look at what iron deficiency is. If we can agree on a definition of anemia, that aside from iron, anemia is a deficiency of red cells, too little hemoglobin, red cells that die too young or are discolored, or possess an abnormal shape, if we can agree on that, we'll say anemia is widespread.

Now to define iron deficiency, we look at the normal limits as described by laboratories. "Normal" limits vary from lab to lab. Let's remember that once iron gets into the body, it is not excreted. The body does shed one milligram or for a woman in reproductive years, an average of one and a half milligram every day. This loss is from hair, fingernails and other detritus. Therefore, to replace that daily loss, the amount required is one to one and a half milligram. This is the way a normal metabolism for iron works.

Jerome Sullivan among others believes the normal iron limits need to be lowered. If your numbers fall below the artificially high levels, you'll automatically be labeled as iron deficient.

Physicians need to be retaught that hemoglobin is not iron. They are two different things. The confusion that low hemoglobin means low iron is so well entrenched that some doctors can't shake off the error. A reader of this book already knows that a woman with low hemoglobin can still be dying of excess iron.

Anemia has many causes. One most common, an iron loading anemia comes about when iron is detoured away from hemoglobin and is redirected into storage.

A study reported in the February 1999; 340:409-17 issue of New England of Journal of Medicine described 838 Canadian patients who were divided into two groups. The study was designed to show rates of death from all causes and whether blood transfusions following surgery is being overused.

One group (418) was transfused when hemoglobin fell below seven, and the second group (420) was transfused when hemoglobin fell below ten. The result was what we have long known, that replacement blood is quickly made when food is eaten.

The study shows that the group not given blood before hemoglobin dropped to seven enjoyed better survival than those transfused unnecessarily to maintain hemoglobin at ten. The difference was 22.2 percent versus 28.1 percent. Conclusion: a restrictive policy on post-op transfusion is at least as effective and possibly superior to the liberal policy. The benefit, of course, was not the low hemoglobin, but the absence of unnecessary excess iron.

In a high malaria area of Gambia two matched groups were fed supplements of iron, thiamine, riboflavin and vitamin C. The conclusion of the study (Trans R. Soc Trop Med Hyg 1987; 81(2)286-91) was that "nutritional intervention may have adverse effects on malaria." An increased incidence of parasites was found in the supplemented group, again suggesting that the offending supplements were the iron together with vitamin C.

Two billion people in the world are iron deficient? Change the normal levels. Measure iron not just hemoglobin. Get rid of their parasites. Find their cancers. Discover where they are losing daily blood.

The person whose food contains less than the needed one milligram a day is on a starvation diet and it's for sure that many other nutrients are also lacking.

More than one and a half million Americans are estimated to be slowly absorbing fatal amounts of iron from their food. This does not count the thirteen percent of the population with the single gene who self medicates with iron, multivitamins and vitamin C or who abuse alcohol. Altogether forty-two million may be affected, counting the newly estimated gene prevalence in Irish and African-Americans.

These people are unaware of their peril. There is no hope for them without prompt action to detect, then remove their excess iron stores. Delayed or missed diagnosis condemns the individual to much body destruction and death.

Awareness is the key. An old Italian proverb goes, "Chi non cerca, non trova." He who doesn't look, doesn't find. If iron is not thought of, it will not be looked for. If it is not looked for, it will not be found.

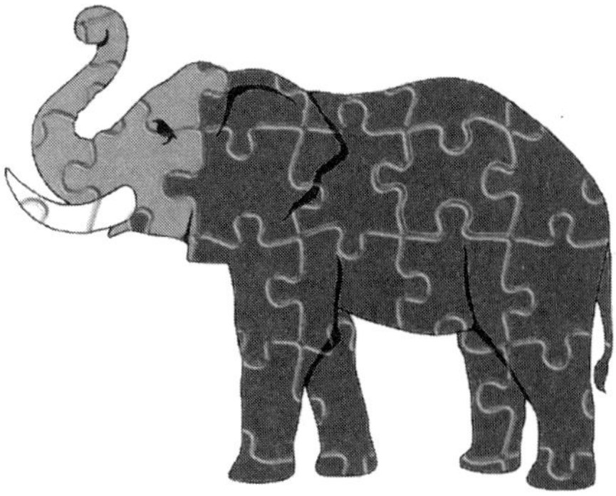

Part 6

"Is there a treatment?"

Chapter 17

The Good News/Bad News Disease

When you tell your family you just found out you have a dreadful disease, the first thing they'll say is, "Can it be treated?"

Hemochromatosis offers one major difference from other terrible diseases. Hemochromatosis is treatable — when detected in time. That's the good news. The other good news is that early detection requires only awareness. Suspect iron, look for it, find it.

Leeches and bloodletting in barber chairs have become antiquated medical curiosities. Get ready for another shock: bleeding is the way to unload iron. Remember, for all practical purposes, iron has no exit from the body except through blood loss.

Blood, the sanguine river of life. It's good to have. It goes where you go, warms you and gives your heart something to pump. Don't let anyone ever describe you as bloodless. They can say you are blooded, and red, blue, hot, even cold — blooded and you'll take it as a compliment.

I watched my blood going down the tube in a thin red stream. It was my sixteenth phlebotomy. Ironic. Years of effort to build an adequate supply, increase the number of red cells, make them redder, encourage them to longer life, improve their hemoglobin content, load them with iron, all down the tube.

Patients have to make an adjustment when they learn of the treatment. It's hard to get used to the idea. But try comparing it to other types of treatment. Compare it to diseases that offer no treatment.

The Archives of Internal Medicine features a section titled "Certain Things Physicians Do." Purpose of the section is described in the heading. "Some customs of practice and prescription outlive their usefulness. Others fall into disuse for no good reason. Others are traditional without a sound basis — historical or contemporary. This feature of the Archives is dedicated to clearing away stumps and underbrush and encouraging a healthy proliferation of neglected good ideas."

One good idea, as it turns out, that fell by the wayside, is bloodletting in certain conditions. In polycythemia, a disorder of excessive red blood cells, bleeding relieves the excess.

In iron overload, excessive iron stores can gradually be unloaded by blood removal.

Pharmacies used to keep bowls of water with leeches on their counters. The worm fastens on the skin and sucks blood, using its three jaws, removing about one-half ounce. A patient needed several leeches to accomplish the job. It is said that Galen, the physician of antiquity, cut off the leeches' tails so the blood could run out and more could be removed by each creature.

An iron overloaded hermit with a wish for do-it-yourself therapy might try raising the worms. I'm told that leeches are indeed used in some surgeries. A leech applied to the hand undergoing surgery will prevent swelling that would hinder the recovery.

During the Twentieth Century hemochromatosis was usually diagnosed after death, that is, if it was recognized at all. The disease was considered to be a novelty and it was believed to be untreatable.

In the winter of 1946 a physician in New Orleans found advanced hemochromatosis in his sixty-seven-year-old patient, a woman. William D. Davis, MD, practiced at Ochsner Clinic. Davis discussed his case with his associate, William Arrowsmith, MD. The pair realized that unless they could remove the excess iron, the patient was facing certain death.

The doctors held long discussions. Did iron have any other way out of the body except through blood loss? No. What about bleeding the patient? Would removing blood unload iron? Could the patient be saved? You can imagine the courage it took in 1946 to revive a medical practice that had been misused in the past and was historically discredited. But it was this patient's only hope of surviving.

"It seemed disarmingly simple," says Davis, now retired, "to attempt to force her to use her tissue iron to manufacture hemoglobin and red blood cells." He ordered the bleeding.

The patient's first phlebotomy was performed in Touro Infirmary on March 23, 1947. It may now be regarded as a landmark date. Millions of subsequent patients can be grateful. On that date five hundred milliliters of blood was removed from the patient. Phlebotomists repeated the procedure on subsequent days until the patient showed a hemoglobin of ten grams and hematocrit of about 30 percent.

After three weeks the patient reported less pain and increased strength and well being. Hemoglobin and hematocrit rose as iron was mobilized out of tissue storage. Despite her distaste for the procedure, the woman continued treatment until 1949. By that time forty liters of blood had been removed. Improvement in the woman's well being was spectacular.

Davis told a physician friend in a northern state about this experience, and shortly afterward the physician diagnosed hemochromatosis in another doctor. The patient insisted on removing a liter of blood and he noted immediate relief from abdominal pain of many months. After a phlebotomy program that took one hundred liters of blood and fifty grams of iron over three and a half years, the patient returned to full time practice.

Other successes followed.

A forty-seven-year-old Texas osteopath had been suffering fatigue, weakness, loss of libido and potency and he had a very large liver and spleen. He was phlebotomized of eighteen quarts in eighteen weeks. He described himself at that time as the picture of health. When last heard from he was in remarkably good health at age eighty-four.

Some of the patients treated by these two doctors are still thriving.

Davis and Arrowsmith were the pioneers in phlebotomy therapy that has changed the outlook from invariably fatal to easily treatable - for those whose excess iron is discovered early.

An attempt had been made in 1942 to remove excess iron by intermittent heavy bleeding, as reported by Balfour and Hahn. However treatment was discontinued. It had been well established by the 1930s that human beings lack a mechanism for excreting iron. It was beginning to dawn on a few doctors that iron's only way out was through bleeding.

Arrowsmith attended IOD's First Symposium in 1983 in New Orleans. Several of his patients from the 1950s were also in the audience. Arrowsmith said he found it interesting to have a chance to talk with doctors from various fields along with experts and patients.

"It has been most gratifying to see the prompt increase in well being and strength in those patients successfully phlebotomized," says Davis, "and to see the objective evidence of liver disease and diabetes improve or disappear in many instances." Davis found it remarkable that "the common complaint of abdominal pain ... disappeared rapidly."

"The treatment of hemochromatosis by repeated phlebotomy has everything to commend it," writes Crosby [Arch Intern Med - Vol 146 Oct 1986].

Crosby says he was refused permission in 1952 to treat a patient whose hepatology consultant would not agree. At a medical meeting in 1958, where the method was discussed, someone in the audience shouted, "Barbarism!"

The medical community has been slow to appreciate the technique, but since 1955 phlebotomy therapy gradually became the accepted life-saving treatment for hemochromatosis.

"Without phlebotomy," said John L. Gollan MD, PhD, "expect five year survival to be only about twenty percent for patients with symptomatic primary hemochromatosis." [Patient Care, Sept. 30, 1982].

The treatment seems drastic to patients and to some physicians.

They should keep in mind, however, that while iron is being removed, slowly, by phlebotomy, there's still plenty in the body to do its dirty work. When they use excuses to avoid bleeding: age, heart disease, low weight and so forth, what they are saying is that the patient is not treatable. In view of the consequences of untreated hemochromatosis, it is not defensible to put off therapy. Lack of understanding about iron leads to exaggerated concern when there's any blood loss. It's common practice to order blood transfusions following many types of surgery, although the human body has the power to make replacement blood fairly rapidly. When occasional patients refuse transfusions, they are then given prescriptions for iron! At the very least this shows a lack of understanding of possible consequences.

If the doctor is timid, the patient is more so.

A Florida woman's liver biopsy showed an iron burden of grade two out of a range of zero to four plus. She suffered no symptoms and she didn't like the idea of frequent bloodlettings. Her doctor was willing to go along with her wishes. "Very well, we'll take a unit of blood and wait two months and make some more tests." Hard to believe, but such stories come to IOD's attention too often. What will happen is that the patient will gradually develop the symptoms to satisfy the diagnosis and then perhaps she will agree to treatment. Her doctor will feel more secure then also.

Ironically, by holding onto their precious blood, such patients with the good fortune of receiving an early diagnosis are throwing away their chance of avoiding complications. The diagnoses are wasted. Diagnosis alone does not save the life. Timid treatment does not work. Vigorous treatment does work.

In a luckier case in another part of Florida a man, informed of the treatment being proposed told his doctor, "You can go to hell." The doctor tapped his finger on the man's chest and replied, "You're going to die." The patient thought it over and agreed.

Other patients are highly motivated, but can't find knowledgeable doctors to order proper treatment.

It's possible to become too anemic to continue treatment although the iron is not all cleaned out. Crosby wrote an article offering help. He wrote, "When almost all of the abnormal storage iron has been removed ... from patients ... I have from time to time encountered a refractory problem. The problem is this: The patient does not recover from the mild anemia after phlebotomy. This is not from lack of iron: serum ferritin levels indicate the persistence of storage iron. Not only does the hematocrit not recover ... but the patient feels wretchedly debilitated. Even a small phlebotomy makes him feel worse.

"Knowing that the male hormone, testosterone, stimulates the marrow to produce red blood cells, I have prescribed depotestosterone for men when this syndrome occurred. They have been promptly improved. One man's hematocrit, for example, went from 38 percent to 45 percent in two weeks, and his disability vanished almost immediately.

"I have proposed testosterone treatment to several women who gracefully declined, preferring fatigue to a moustache. It is possible that Megace might be useful, but I've no experience of it. It does improve hemoglobin levels in women with metastatic breast cancer who have the anemia of chronic disease.

"Erythropoietin has recently been released by the FDA for use in patients with the anemia of renal disease. Erythropoietin is the hormone which naturally stimulates the marrow to produce red blood cells, and the kidney is its source.

"I know of one woman with hemochromatosis who suffered from the debilitating syndrome well before all the abnormal storage iron had been mobilized and removed. She could not tolerate even a half-size phlebotomy. Erythropoietin injections three times a week promptly improved her hematocrit and her well being, and permitted the last of the abnormal iron to be removed.

"Of course one robin doesn't make a spring, and one patient's good response doesn't mean that erythropoietin can help everyone. But erythropoietin is practically devoid of side effects, and it may be worth a trial in women with this syndrome.

"Why is it necessary to get rid of those last iron nuggets in the liver? We don't know which of the deposits ... cause the complications. Until we do, it seems prudent to clean out all of it."

The blood bank is the place to go for treatment. Blood banks do not take blood from donors more often than about every 56 days, so it is necessary to present a prescription from a physician. You need a physician's permission for treatment. The prescription should read: This hemochromatosis patient requires weekly or twice weekly phlebotomies. Before each one his/her hematocrit must be _____. He sets a cut off. Many doctors are more concerned about anemia than iron. They set the cut off too high and make the patient untreatable. A little anemia will not kill you. A hematocrit of between 30 and 35 is reasonable. Since I started out anemic, I insisted on a cut off of 28.

Virgil F Fairbanks MD of the Mayo Clinic wrote about a case that was treated intensively. The young man suffered B-thalassemia minor, an iron-loading anemia and severe hemochromatosis. At age ten he was treated with large doses of oral iron daily. By age 24 he had developed many of the signs and symptoms: severe fatigues, joint and abdominal pain, shortness of breath, palpitations and darkening of his skin, among others.

Fairbanks reported that his blood sugar was elevated and liver enzymes were very high. Saturation was nearly 100 percent and serum ferritin was an astounding 72,500. The patient had advanced cirrhosis.

"What to do? Obviously have him stop taking iron pills. But that would not be enough. Because of the thalassemia he was anemic. His hemoglobin was 8.8. Normal would be in the range of 14 to 18. "In spite of the anemia he was treated vigorously by phlebotomy.

"Today, 16 years later, he is doing well. He has no abdominal or joint pain. He is not short of breath. He does not have palpitations. He is not hyperpigmented, and his liver and spleen are of normal size. He does not have diabetes. His liver is functioning normally, and his liver enzymes are normal."

Some physicians do the bloodletting in their offices. If you agree to that, don't let them use a glass jug. The vacuum will collapse the veins and sometimes lead to more than one stick. You need to protect the veins. It has been suggested that you rub the scar tissue with vitamin E oil. Some patients take an aspirin before the procedure to make the blood flow easier.

A patient in Arvada, Colorado wrote to us that he is doing better now, using a 21 gauge needle. No more vein spasms. There's no reason to use larger needles. Blood banks should be willing to do this for you.

Pat of Yonkers, New York suggested a way to have pain free phlebotomies. She sprays her arm with ethyl choride to numb the puncture spot.

We believe blood banks do it better. It's all they do and they are good at it. Blood banks are always crying for blood. It is rumored that they import blood from other countries. They accept any donor off the street, after putting the blood through ten tests. We have urged blood banks to accept hemochromatosis patients as donors, but they have resisted stubbornly.

It infuriates patients to have to spend large sums for phlebotomies. Some blood banks charge up to $400 for each phlebotomy, and some physicians require the patient to make an office visit or have the procedure done at a hospital.

An expose in *US News and World Report, Sept 1 1997,* explained that blood banks generate roughly $200 million in gross revenues by charging these patients and discarding their blood. The blood is not iron-loaded. Iron is in storage in organs and tissue. The blood is in fact perfectly good and a bit superior in that it has younger, newer red cells that will last longer in those receiving it. This is because these people give much more often.

Again the irony is, as we point out to the blood banking community, if they think this blood is bad, they are using it, because most iron overloaded people are not diagnosed. Blood banks do not measure iron. They don't know the iron status of any donor.

It looks as if blood banks are not willing to give up this increasing supply of money. Increasing because as doctors become more aware they are beginning to diagnose more and more.

The article said, "The waste of blood has enraged many hematologists." Dr Stephen Strum was quoted as saying, "It's an ethical and medical travesty." Dr James Kushner said, "They're ignoring a huge pool of healthy donors that could wipe out the shortages overnight."

It is true too, as Corwin Edwards MD has pointed out that hemochromatosis patients are the "most motivated, medically scrutinized, on time donors to be found."

Blood banking's excuse is that patients are not giving "altruistically."

"It's big business, a big scandal and a black mark on blood bankers," says Victor Herbert.

The article quoted a patient in Portland, Oregon, who admitted he travels from blood bank to blood bank, not mentioning his disease. However since the article was printed, the man told us the blood banks refuse to accept him.

Walter in New England was told his blood is dangerous for donating. He asked if they tested for iron. No. "Well," he said, "most people with iron overload are not diagnosed." He said, "Is the public aware that the Red Cross accepts dangerous blood?"

"I could almost do it myself," declared a young Alabama man. He was thinking about training his wife to do it. "I think I could," she said. "Why not?" said her husband. "Where I work there are two women who were secretaries one day and phlebotomists the next. It can't be that hard."

Patients see anonymous donors come in off the street, offer their blood and have it accepted as donor blood. A percentage of these people may well have undiagnosed hemochromatosis. Why, patients ask, should they be penalized for being correctly diagnosed?

Often a patient will ask why the blood banks don't use their blood. K. Sigvaard Olsson MD PhD, of Molndal, Sweden, wrote to IOD that he agrees that hemochromatosis patients' blood should be accepted as donor blood. Many Swedish blood banks offer routine lab tests to determine serum iron, TIBC or serum ferritin, Olsson wrote. Iron overloaded subjects are thereby detected while still healthy. Swedish blood banks do accept these people as donors. "Their blood is actually better," says Olsson, (not because it has high iron; the iron is in organs and tissue) "because it contains more young red cells that last longer in the recipient." The recipient can then get along with fewer transfusions. Olsson concludes, "Who should be paid?" It's a case where an iron-overloaded patient can help lessen iron overload in an individual with iron-loading anemia.

The reason iron overloaded patients have younger red cells is simply that by bleeding weekly and making replacement blood weekly, their red cell population is constantly turning over and the cells are younger.

A Chicago blood bank used to call Alan in the middle of the night to give arm-to-arm transfusion because his blood was "rare." It was in demand. That was before hemochromatosis was discovered. Not before he had the condition - before it was found. When officials didn't know he was iron-overloaded, they held Alan's blood in high regard. If the blood bank had given the routine tests Olsson reports are given in Sweden, it could have saved Alan considerable anguish. He visited doctors including specialists at three clinics for eight years. Their diagnoses: "You're depressed." "Your job is causing stress." "Eczema." Finally a correct diagnosis was made.

Now Alan still goes to the blood bank, but now he pays for the privilege. That same blood bank is undoubtedly using blood unknowingly from a number of donors whose high iron is not yet discovered. Genetic estimates for the disease suggest that with Chicago's almost three million population, there are 15,000 people who carry the double gene. And what about the other thirteen percent, those who carry the single gene? Those 390,000? Many are taking iron, vitamin C and using alcohol excessively. Most of those affected are unaware of their danger. The blood banks don't know who they are.

"It is indeed a shame," writes Alice from Michigan, "for the blood bank to be crying for blood when all they ever do ... is take our blood and then right in front of our eyes they throw it in the waste basket!" They say they can't use it, she says, and adds, "This is really hard to believe."

In answer to a patient's question at a symposium, Walter G. Frey III, MD, said, "You have to deal with a bureaucratic structure. They may be uninfluenceable. We happen to be lucky to have a reaasonable person to deal with. One of the reasons we have been successful up there (Vermont) is one of our patients was a go-getter. He made himself the lay head of the Vermont-New Hampshire Red Cross program and got what he wanted. That's one way of influencing bureaucratic holdups and that's all it is."

IOD offered a pool of hemochromatosis donor blood to the nation's blood banks in September 1983 during a blood bank crisis and blood shortage caused by the AIDs scare. I said, "We don't give more cheerfully, but we do give more often."

There were no takers.

At a meeting in Dusseldorf I called on blood banks to not only accept and use the blood of these patients, I told blood banks that they are morally obligated to test for iron and help identify patients. They have the blood. They have the labs. They already do at least ten tests.

On April 30, 1999 the Advisory Committee on Blood Safety and Availability voted to "eliminate the barriers to using" donor blood from individuals with hemochromatosis. Blood banks will have to go along with that because of the constant shortages of blood and since they must begin to recognize they are already using blood from people who do have too much iron, but are not diagnosed.

This will be a great benefit to health care. Free treatment for a common condition. However, the only patients who will benefit will be those who are diagnosed early, before liver damage that will result in elevated liver enzymes, people who are not taking strong medication for diabetes, arthritis, heart disease or cancer. In other words, the diagnosis must be made before body damage.

The blood must be perfectly good to be usable.

From Michigan: "I have anemia that is progressing toward aplastic and to date have received 157 units of red cells. I have not had any serious problems with iron overload yet but will eventually." (What are they waiting for?!)

For patients who can't be bled because they are severely anemic, chelation is available. Advances in chelation technique that infuses the drug, Desferal, over a twelve hour period instead of the former injection, now give better results.

Newest techniques deliver the drug by implanted pump. Though expensive and not convenient, chelation will prolong the life of a frequently transfused patient.

An Orlando woman had long suffered anemia for which she

was given Trinsicon. It was eventually determined that her anemia was thalassemia minor, an anemia that is iron loading.

Edwards wrote a fascinating paper in **BLOOD,** in which he discussed the problem of patients with genes for both thalassemia and hemochromatosis. The anemia of thalassemia is not an iron deficiency. Iron should not be administered. But the Orlando woman had acquired hemochromatosis or had developed it genetically with thalassemia. The woman's next problem was to find a physician to order phlebotomies. Bleeding an anemic patient imposed too much strain on the physician's understanding of iron. With a hematocrit range of 35 to 39 percent, the anemia was not too severe to rule out bleeding. If that were true, many of us would not still be here.

The woman spent two years of indecision, sometimes searching for a doctor and other times being lulled by doctors' judgments that she should not be bled, that she was in effect untreatable. Meanwhile the patient developed severe heart and liver disease.

Fairbanks tells of ordering regular phlebotomies on a similar patient. He has no reluctance to do it when the patient's hemoglobin is ten g/dl, or hematocrit is at least 30 percent. In fact, recall the patient with more than 70,000 ferritin and a hemoglobin of 8.8. Without vigorous therapy that patient could not have lived.

Georg Kontoghiorghes MD, in London, has reported in The Lancet on a new approach he and colleagues are developing to chelate iron. He reported details of the chemical components and said that urinary iron was increased several times over other chelators, and that the excretion of copper, zinc, magnesium and calcium was not affected. [April 6, 1985]. The compound is still in the testing stage.

When patients are too anemic to be bled, as was Dot in Georgia, they must be given the support of chelation therapy. Paul Cutler, MD, at Niagara Falls, New York, often combines chelation with phlebotomy to speed the exit of iron.

Cutler spoke at IOD's 17th Annual Symposium. He told of four patients who were on a heart transplant list. After Cutler initiated intensive treatment, including chelation with Desferal, those patients improved enough not to need the transplants.

Cutler told of one diabetic patient who was preparing for leg amputation. Cutler was able to save the leg by using Desferal. He has also reported success treating psychiatric patients.

The dilemma of severe anemia and the increasing accumulation of iron stores is like being on a runaway train headed for collision with another runaway train from the opposite direction. When the collision came, Dot died.

The only brakes that can be applied to the hemochromatosis train in severe anemia, is a chelating drug to slow down iron accumulation. The chelation drug must be started early. Later is too late.

Victor Herbert MD, JD, stood with his hands on hips, making his point at IOD's 14th Annual Symposium in St Louis. He told of a half dozen kids who died from massive doses of vitamin C while being chelated. They had thalassemia and were too anemic to be bled. Doctors then realized that too much vitamin C pushed iron into the heart. Herbert says, "No over the counter vitamin C." The vitamin not only enhances the absorption of iron, but it mobilizes iron around the body and makes it more toxic. The public keeps being told to take antioxidants. But in the presence of iron these become *pro*oxidants.

A Texas man in his late twenties was told he had too much iron. Doctors advised him to cut down on foods with iron and perhaps give a pint of blood every three months or so. They told him if he didn't take care of the situation he would have a dreadful disease. Bad advice! Cutting down on high iron foods is no help as there is no way you can design a healthy diet if you delete the many foods with high iron. Giving blood only every three months is less often than regular blood donors. Bad advice!

Many patients and their doctors hit a "plateau" of indecision about when to cease intensive therapy. Corwin Edwards recommends twice weekly phlebotomies until the hematocrit stays at 33 percent for two consecutive phlebotomies. At this point suspend blood removals for one to three months.

Newest information says take the ferritin to below ten or even zero. Storage iron is not necessary. At that point you need to design a maintenance program, which is experimental the first year because everyone is different. Try a schedule of giving blood every two or three or four months. At the end of the year measure the ferritin to see if it is still below ten. Adjust the schedule as needed. Do this every year. You no longer need to measure the saturation. You are not trying to keep hematocrit low, only ferritin.

Maintenance therapy is usually scheduled for every two months for men, Edwards said, and every three or four months for women. Allow the hematocrit to become normal. The transferrin saturation may rise, and may remain high despite iron depletion. It cannot be used as an indicator of the need for phlebotomy, but the serum ferritin is not allowed to rise.

Crosby spoke at IOD's Second Annual Symposium, describing that the way phlebotomy works is that it creates a mild anemia that stimulates the bone marrow to make replacement blood, thereby withdrawing iron from stores. He told of a case he had treated years before.

Crosby had increased phlebotomies to twice and thrice weekly trying to get the patient's hematocrit below 40 percent. Finally he had the patient on a five-a-week schedule, which was maintained for six weeks before frequency had to be cut back.

The thing to remember about treatment is the faster you get the iron out, the better for the patient. Early detection and vigorous treatment.

Intensive treatment made a difference in Jennifer's outcome. It was the first reported case of restoring fertility by getting rid of iron vigorously.

An emergency call came to IOD offices one day from a co-worker of a forty-two-year-old man. He had been diagnosed a year earlier, never treated. Now he was in congestive heart failure, and his office mates wanted information rushed to them about a knowledgeable physician in their area. It was too late.

Mrs. C in Los Altos, California was concerned about her brother. He was being treated with one unit of blood drawn each month. His sister had read that phlebotomies should be more frequent.

A Florida school worker's doctor told her that she would need to have blood drawn about three times a year. The patient had tested with 100 percent saturation.

Marguerite of Bloomingdale, Illinois was identified as having hemochromatosis, but her doctor, she says, "has little or no knowledge of the disease ... he sees no need for any particular treatment."

Dixie of Omaha, Nebraska is concerned about her husband. "We were told he has this disease, but they seem to be doing nothing about it because they don't seem to know what or how to treat it. All the medical books I look into don't even have it listed."

Bill of Fort Worth, Texas says, "I feel better than I have ever felt in my life." He received a correct diagnosis and aggressive treatment. On his way to a Caribbean cruise he stopped off at the Palm Beach Blood Bank for a treatment, not willing to miss therapy. That's dedication. He would like to give hope to people who are victims of this disease. "You can live with hemochromatosis," he says, "and if you find it early enough, there's hope."

Barbara's husband, George, is serving in the United States military. He started suffering vague pain in his knees, back and chest. The alert hematologist evaluating him did a thorough work-up and found both thalassemia and hemochromatosis. Correct treatment promptly began, but physicians ignored the pain and said it was "unrelated." George feels a sense of defeat by the doctors' unconcern with his discomforts.

A correctional institutional inmate was refused treatment for his hemochromatosis. We do not know his crime or his sentence. On his behalf we wrote to the medical director of the facility. Ironically many people in the state where he is incarcerated are running around untreated, undiagnosed. But, as we wrote the doctor, these other citizens at least do theoretically have a choice. Without treatment this man is on death row.

To help patients understand the gravity of the condition and to motivate them to get rid of the iron vigorously, Felitti and Kaiser gives each patient a video tape and a copy of *The Iron Elephant.* "We buy that book by the case," he said.

The iron chelator has been used in other diseases to reduce iron levels to help treatment of the disease: Parkinson's, Huntington's chorea, Alzheimer's, tardine dyskinesia, spastic paraplegia and Hallervorden-Spatz. Iron removal also helps in treating hepatitis and cancer (unless the cancer has already used up the iron). A study in Hokuriku University at Kanazawa Japan showed that "iron deficiency is unfavorable for malignant growth," in other words favorable to inhibit cancer.

Iron-depleting agents have been given directly to bladder cancer cells and were found effective in reducing tumor growth.

The arthritic pain associated with iron overload remains a difficult burden for the patient. Frederick Dietz MD, Rockford Illinois, rheumatologist, speaking at IOD's Fifth Symposium, said that some of his patients report improvement with water beds - "the best thing that ever happened" - but that others are not helped.

Finding a doctor who will permit correct treatment can be difficult. IOD has instituted a physician referral registry, a directory of physicians still thinly spread across the country and in a few other countries. Patients feel extreme gratitude for these doctors who are knowledgeable and caring. Luckily the numbers of such good doctors are increasing rapidly. But still many areas are without physicians who are up-to-date about iron. An alternative for the patient would be to find a doctor willing to consult with authorities. Many experts are generous and gladly willing to help.

Mr. H was treated in Hillsboro, Ohio. After about 96 bloodlettings he regained lost weight. He had dropped from 185 to 135. Now he weighs in at 170 and says, "I feel good, working every day twelve to fourteen hours, only need three to four hours sleep, can eat almost anything."

And what about diet? One of the first questions that comes to IOD is, "Can you give me a diet?" The answer is no. There is no healthy iron-free diet. You already realize this if you have been struggling to devise such a diet and found it impossible. Your dietitian tried and couldn't do it. Iron is in virtually everything. Dietitians call us. "What do you recommend?"

We do not recommend an iron poor diet. The foods high in iron are the same foods that include the other nutrients essential to repair your body. Deleting high iron foods means you are deleting necessary nutrients.

Your main goal is to prevent liver cancer. You do this first by unloading excess iron as fast as possible. While your liver is busy trying to heal, give it a break. The liver yearns for a large variety of fresh fruits, fresh vegetables, grains and other natural, not processed foods. Your liver prefers small portions.

When you do occasionally serve products such as cereals and canned or frozen foods, be sure to read the labels. Food companies add iron to these products, but they must reveal the amount on the label.

"Cereal killers" are among the worst. You'll read that Total, for example, gives 100 percent of your "daily allowance for iron." And remember, the daily allowance is set too high. Return the Total to the store shelf.

Most patients compromise by eating shredded wheat or oatmeal.

In the past we suggested that it was a good idea to drink tea with meals. Tea helps to inhibit iron absorption. We no longer recommend this. It doesn't make that much difference, and you may be lulled into belicving you are accomplishing more than is the case. Drink tea if you like it.

At the same time we used to suggest that you save orange juice and other vitamin C foods to enjoy between meals, since vitamin C enhances iron absorption. Now we have a better understanding that there is very little to be done to avoid absorbing iron. The simple solution is to know your level and keep the excess unloaded.

A special warning about vitamin C taken in pill form is required here. When the vitamin has been reduced in this way it becomes toxic, much more so in the presence of iron. When vitamin C appears naturally in a variety of food it does not have this effect. But in pill form the vitamin attaches itself to iron and becomes prooxidant instead of antioxidant. It can mobilize the iron into the heart muscle, where it can do a great deal of damage.

Patients sometimes feel that if they take multivitamins without iron, no harm is done. A B complex, in fact, may help in some cases, but be sure to avoid vitamin C additives.

No matter what report you were given on the condition of your liver, you should assume some liver damage. This damage does not show up on the liver enzyme tests until the injury has become considerable. Therefore you must avoid alcohol. Alcohol is toxic to damaged liver cells. You do not want your liver to endure the combination of iron and alcohol.

After the iron is totally cleaned out, after there are no more symptoms from liver injury, such as abdominal pain, diarrhea, mental confusion and so on, resume alcohol use with extreme moderation. A drink on your birthday. Very, very slowly at first and for a long time.

By now we all know what a healthy diet is. The pyramid, big at the bottom with grains, narrowing slightly with the wonderful fresh fruits and vegetables, narrowing a little more with meat, eggs and dairy, leaving desserts to perch on the top point. Give this pyramid of delicious food daily to your liver in small portions. Enjoy!

Art Buchwald once said that sexual anorexia is caused by Monday Night Football. That's a good possibility. However the most frequently missed cause of impotence or loss of libido is an excess of iron.

Too few laughs come into IOD offices. But one day we had a chuckle that lasted all day. Every year we observe Iron Overload Awareness Week in September. We mail our publications to the governors to keep them informed and ask them to sign proclamations. There are off-shore possessions and protectorates of the U.S. that were left out of our mailing, until by chance, we happened to mail January-February 1986 *Ironic Blood* to some island governors. By purest accident the story of that issue was how to improve testicular function.

Here's the scene. The island governor who had never heard of us or iron overload or the problems of testicles associated with hemochromatosis gets this advice in the mail on how to improve testicular function. We hadn't meant anything personal ... we weren't suggesting that anyone needed his testicular function improved. That day a letter came from the governor's press aide ..."I want you to know that in no way did I ever subscribe to your newsletter for the governor or myself. I am not interested, nor has the governor in receiving future issues, so take his name off your mailing list ... I have a favor to ask of you. Can you please send me a copy of the subscription allegedly from me so I could find out just who the hell made that application?"

There are patients who very much appreciate the work being

done to preserve or restore testicular function. Arturo R. Rolla, MD, wrote the article that went to the governor. He said that traditional medical teaching has been that the testis affected by hemochromatosis will never improve with treatment. "Never say never," said Rolla. He offered a "new ray of hope" from the University of Utah Medical School. Edwards and his colleagues followed very closely for many years a group of forty-one males with hemochromatosis. Five of the patients were found to have moderate to severe testicular and/or pituitary damage. After prolonged treatment with blood withdrawals, two of the five noted an improvement in their sex drive and increased growth of body hair. The improvement was confirmed by careful measurement of testosterone (male hormone).

Injections directly into the penis have restored virility for one IOD member in Louisiana. He reported the success to benefit others. The drug injected was Papaverine. The same man had found no relief with testosterone.

Crosby recommends medicinal help. "For endocrine-deficiency states," he says, "replacement therapy is essential. Insulin is needed for the control of most diabetes. Steroids are also essential to treat the postmenopausal state, especially in amenorrheal young women, and in impotent young men. Testosterone may also increase the erythropoietic activity of the marrow, permitting more frequent phlebotomy." Another aid to continuing phlebotomies when the hematocrit drops too low for bleeding, is erythropioetin, which will stimulate the marrow. Women prefer it to testosterone.

Instead of trying for an iron poor diet, try to give your liver the freshest of produce type foods, fruits and vegetables..

Even with collapsed or damaged veins, phlebotomies can often be continued. Esther of Graham, Washington, said the Hickman catheter is a godsend. The device is installed under the skin and into a major vein, eliminating the need for the periodic sticking of needles.

Barry Skikne, MD, has helped his patients at University of Kansas by modifying the usual phlebotomy methods of a large gauge needle and vacuum bag. He says that vacuum bags can cause too much pressure that can irritate or collapse the vein.

Instead Skikne uses 19 or 21 gauge needles. He withdraws the blood slowly by two large syringes. He has eliminated all problems with this technique.

The diabetes encountered is treated the same as any diabetes, except of course the underlying iron must be removed. Often with early detection and aggressive treatment, the diabetes will improve significantly. The diabetes can also become less insulin-dependent and much easier to manage.

Iron overloaded patients with diabetes do appear to require more insulin, and often the diabetes is more insulin-dependent, unless the iron is unloaded early. With proper phlebotomy treatment, fifty percent of the patients will see an improvement in the diabetes.

Donald Ritt, MD, suggested a way to deal with the mental changes caused by liver damage. He was speaking to patients in 1982 at a meeting of American Liver Foundation, held in Chicago. Limiting protein may help. The patient should experiment to find the maximum amount of protein his liver can handle without problems.

Hospital workers in Australia "blamed themselves," a woman said, after her husband lapsed into unconsciousness that lasted for twenty-four hours. The patient was iron overloaded and was taken to hospital with liver failure. Hospital personnel admitted "they gave him too much protein." Too much protein presented to a damaged liver allows ammonia to back up into the brain.

Another word before we leave the subject of treatment. It has been recommended that iron overloaded patients avoid eating or handling raw seafood. If after being at the seashore they see signs of blood poisoning, fever and shock or skin infection, they should alert their doctors to their special vulnerability to the Vibrio vulnificus found in many waters..

If you do become infected, you need prompt treatment with penicillin or tetracycline. With plenty of iron to feed the Vibrio, proliferation can develop fast, with death within forty-eight hours.

I repeat this can be a "good news" condition. Carolyn in Pittsburgh dropped her ferritin from 4,000 to 11. She said,"It's great to feel alive again." It's hard to imagine a disease that is cheaper to diagnose or cheaper to treat - when found early. Yet, miss the diagnosis, neglect the treatment, and iron overload can cost you a fortune as well as your life.

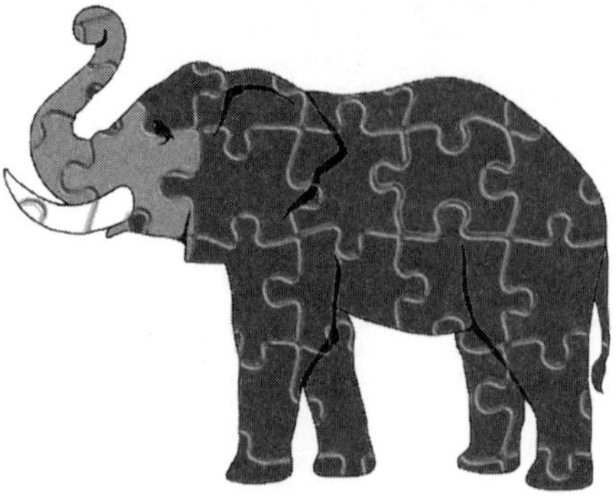

Part 7

"Isn't any research being done?"

Chapter 18

It's Already Getting Better

A hundred years ago when hemochromatosis was found only at autopsy, the disease was considered to be untreatable.

The slow progress during the interval can be blamed on attitude, or lack of awareness. "Research funding is hard to come by," said James C. Barton, MD, in a Birmingham (Alabama) News story by Bob Blalok, "but hemochromatosis will have its day." [Oct. 1, 1985].

Hemochromatosis has become a hot medical subject. Physicians packed the halls for symposiums by IOD for American College of Physicians (1985 and 1986) and for the American Gastroenterological Association (1987) at their annual meetings. At international meetings, sessions on iron overload were well attended in 1988 at International Society of Hematology in Milan, in 1989 at an Update in Australia, in 1991 in Dusseldorf, Germany, again in New York, in St Malo, France and in Sorrento, Italy. A special meeting focusing on iron and HIV was held in Brugge, Belgium as well as several meetings in the U. S. held by the National Institutes of Health and the Centers for Disease Control.

Blood tests are available that measure transferrin saturation and serum ferritin. Liver biopsies can give an accurate picture of the iron status of the liver. With quantitative analysis, you can determine the amount of excess iron to be unloaded. The entire subject has been much simplified. Most physicians now feel that the liver biopsy is not necessary.

Phlebotomy therapy is available. Chelation therapy is available, although it needs further research to become truly satisfactory.

Tissue matching of family members has been available for some time, and for the curious there are now DNA tests. DNA is all right to confirm, but not to rule out the diagnosis. An unknown number of mutations remain to be discovered.

Still tragedies continue. As I write this at the end of a millennium, a phone call interrupts. A woman has been told she has hemochromatosis, but since she is anemic she must take iron three times a day. Her hemoglobin is low! I told her it's her life and her death. She must throw away the iron medicine, and for the anemia she probably needs folic acid ("Oh, I'm getting that") with B12, since they work together and since such deficiency produces iron loading anemia. There has been an odd resistance in the medical profession, and hemochromatosis has not received the attention and prominence it should have. Even physicians well acquainted with the disease think of it as something exotic, "someone else's." A well-respected physician failed to make the diagnosis in his own son.

Doctors think of it as a disease, with symptoms, to be treated, if a diagnosis is established. No. Forget disease. Everybody has iron. The only question is how much do you have and can you get it lower to protect your heart and your liver and your brain and your sex life.

A prosperous Illinois surgeon confided to his golfing partner that he was worried about his wife. They were walking back to the clubhouse. All the top doctors had given her every test they could think of, but she was getting worse every day.

Sam listened sympathetically. His own wife was finally feeling better. She had also had many tests before excess iron was found. At IOD's urging, she had insisted on intensive treatment.

Sam squinted against the sun. "... excruciating abdominal cramping in the middle of the night ... sleeping twelve hour stretches ... forgetfulness ..." Sam stopped walking. "...bruises ... swollen hands ..." Sam hesitated. How do you give medical advice to a doctor? Then, remembering the great difficulty of Janet's diagnosis — it very nearly didn't happen. "Walt —" He couldn't tell whether Walt was paying attention. Oh, well. After all, it could make a difference. Sam took the plunge and told his friend about Janet's experience. He suggested iron testing.

A few weeks later Sam got a call. "What's the name of those tests?"

By then the surgeon's wife was dying in the hospital. Iron tests did reveal hemochromatosis. That word — hemochromatosis — still carries an aura of the exotic, the remote. The disease has an "orphan" quality, not because it is rare, but because it belongs to no one medical specialty. It's too simple, just a metabolic condition.

The need for universal screening is obvious. On January 2 1990 MetPath Laboratories, now Quest, did add the iron panel to their ChemScreen, at IOD's urging. We had exhibited at a meeting of pathologists, where our message was: It's Up To The Labs.

During the first few months MetPath discovered dangerously elevated iron in 100,000 tests. Those patients were being treated by their physicians for everything under the sun, their iron levels unknown. Dying. The patients were dying. Because of MetPath's new test policies many lives were saved.

Harold Bates, MetPath's Director of Scientific Affairs, compiled results in a study that found that:

-Only 16.7 percent of the physicians were aware of the relationship between iron overload and impotence. Twelve cases of low testosterone with low levels of serum luteinizing hormone levels were identified. Transferrin saturation was greater than 50 percent; serum ferritin was greater than 500! Only two of the physicians treating these people were aware that iron overload could lead to gonadotropin deficiency and diminished sexual function. Iron overload is the most overlooked cause of impotence.

-eighty cases of arthritis were identified: 22 males and 58 females. Transferrin saturation was greater than 50 percent; serum ferritin was greater than 500. Only 11.3 percent of their physicians were aware of the relationship between arthropathy and iron overload. Only nine of the eighty doctors understood that iron overload could injure joints and cause arthritis in hands and knees and destroy hips.

-167 cases were identified with a variety of heart problems, 162 males and five females. The damage ranged from congestive cardiomyopathy with bilateral ventricular dilation to pulmonary congestion and peripheral edema. Some suffered arrythmias or nonspecific EKG changes. Physicians ordered serum digoxin, serum procainamide or serum quinidine levels. But transferrin saturations were greater than 50 percent, serum ferritin was more than 500. Only 6.6 percent of cardiologists contacted were aware of the relationship between iron overload and congestive heart failure. Only eleven of the 167 doctors contacted were aware that iron overload damages the heart.

IOD's survey showed that patients are being treated by cardiologists, dermatologists, endocrinologists, family practitioners, general practitioners, gastroenterologists, gynecologists, hematologists, hepatologists, internists, oncologists, rheumatologists, etc. However, any family physician or general practitioner can treat this simple condition.

A few corporations began adding the iron panel to their employee screening. CIBA (now Novartis) in Alabama immediately identified two patients. Presumably early, treatable diagnoses. Costs to test and treat iron overload are nominal. Some labs set the cut off at 62 percent saturation and 450 ferritin. Numbers above that were suspect and required further study. Those numbers are all right if you are willing to miss cases. More practical cut offs are 45 percent on saturation and 150 on ferritin.

In the early 1990s IOD was deluged with mail and phone calls following publication of an article in *Parade Magazine* and in an *Ann Landers* column. The stories were heart breaking. Nobody else had access to those experiences, and we felt urgently impelled to get the information out to the public. Achieving media attention remains as difficult as ever.

We knew too that the medical community needed this information. We participated in as many medical meetings as we could afford. We designed a display with three alternating photos. (1) a sparkling new automobile with the words: **excess iron** (2) photo of a rusted junk yard car with the word: **rusts** (3) photo of bathing beauty emerging from the ocean with the word: **bodies.**

In June 1997 an international gathering of physicians and scientists studying aspects of iron overload gathered in Saint-Malo, France. Serious attention was paid to the many diseases that are affected by excess iron. Alzheimer's, Huntington's chorea, tardine dyskinesia, spastic paraplegia and Hallervorden-Spatz.

Several cancer studies showed iron to be a factor. African iron overload was noted as a risk factor for pulmonary tuberculosis. The odds for TB in subjects with iron overload was 1.7 times the odds in those without.

A study reported from Wake Forest University concluded that delivering iron-depleting agents (gallium) directly to bladder cancer cells was effective in reducing tumor growth.

When Corwin Q. Edwards was a medical student, he says, some interesting things were going on at University of Utah. Some of the researchers, George Cartwright and Wintrobe, were making immense impact on matters of iron, as was William Crosby elsewhere. "I thought hemochromatosis would be an ideal subject," Edwards said, "but some experts persuaded me that it was too rare and I wouldn't have anybody to study. However we soon began seeing patients at the University that led to the family studies." In a family that was dealing with both hemochromatosis and thalassemia, researchers found greatly elevated transferrin saturation in children ages four, five and seven. It has been suggested that in some diseases such as porphyria, the disease may be silent and not expressed unless it is combined with an H gene.

Lack of correct information in some parts of the medical profession continues to create problems. Ruth of Myrtle Creek, Oregon, was told by a physician that hemochromatosis is "handed down to all the male members of the family." Ruth's brother-in-law had died at sixty-four of the disease, discovered too late and treated inadequately, and she was worried about her husband, then sixty-one, already suffering arthritis.

A Florida woman wrote, "We are quite concerned regarding David's condition since the specialist who tested and diagnosed him, did not recommend any treatment whatsoever. He only scheduled him to have another blood workup in six months." Months later she wrote to IOD that her husband had been treated with "two sets of three bleedings each month and will rest a month before going back to his internist for further blood tests." But timid treatment does not work. Only vigorous, intensive treatment works, and proper, adequate treatment makes all the difference.

At the same time we are seeing much improvement. The Hickman catheter, previously mentioned, for example, helps those with problem veins. Esther, for one, is grateful. "The procedure is done with local anesthetic," and it takes about twelve minutes. "It's a piece of cake," Esther said. "I call it my lifeline." A small incision is made in the chest near thc collar bone and the tube is placed into a large blood vessel and guided into place. The other end of the tube is guided under the skin for a few inches and brought out through another small incision on the chest. Esther said,"I thank God for the Hickman catheter."

After six years on the Hickman, Esther switched to a port-a-cath, which is accessed by a needle. "These tubes have kept me going!" she says.

Research is being conducted in Germany, where Wolfgang Stremmel, MD, recently isolated a protein from the intestine, which may be a carrier protein for iron and may be involved in the pathogenesis of increased iron absorption.

— Charleston, South Carolina, VA Medical Center, Jerome L. Sullivan, MD, PhD, was investigating iron depletion, tissue injury and acute inflammation. He has since relocated to University of Florida.

— London, England, The Royal Free Hospital, Georg Kontoghiorghes, MD, is working to develop oral iron chelators. Rabbits are used to demonstrate the effectiveness of a chelating compound, reported in British Journal of Haematology, [1986, 62, 607-613]. Iron excretion was comparable to desferrioxamine. Examination of the urine during the administration of the chelators revealed their high specificity for iron but not for copper, zinc, calcium or magnesium. There was no apparent toxicity. The chelators were administered orally. The first clinical trials were conducted later and were being published in the summer of 1987.

— South Africa. Oral chelators are being tested on humans. There is much hope that these chelators will help children who suffer thalassemia major. The children have been required to endure injections or infusion of chelating drugs.

— Salt Lake City, Utah, University of Utah, Corwin Q. Edwards, MD, and colleagues, conduct family and other studies.

— Molndal, Sweden, K. Sigvard Olsson, MD, conducts screening studies of the population.

— University of North Carolina, James D. Oliver, PhD, the effects of Vibrio vulnificus on iron overloaded patients.

— Porto, Portugal, Maria de Sousa, MD, PhD, studies the effects of excess iron on the immune system and iron's relationship to cancer.

— Gainesville, Florida, Raymond J. Bergeron, PhD, and Richard R. Streiff, MD, are working on developing chelating compounds.

—Johannesburg, South Africa, University of Witwatersrand, Thomas H. Bothwell, MD, investigates a mechanism by which iron is metabolized.

— Cleveland, Ohio, Case Western Reserve University, John Harris, MD, and colleagues, were developing the superconducting quantum-interference-device, the SQUID. At the same university Bruce Bacon, MD, now at St. Louis University, Gary Brittenham, MD, and Anthony Tavill, MD, with colleagues have studied the mechanism of liver damage in rats with chronic iron overload. The rats were iron overloaded by feeding a special diet supplemented with finely divided elemental iron. Workers observed that high hepatic iron concentration produced significant liver damage and scar tissue formation. Massive dietary iron produced higher hepatic iron concentration than iron injection.

Dr. Bacon and colleagues did studies to learn how iron works its damage on liver cells. The investigators prepared sections of rat liver in the test tubes and examined the effects of iron injury. They found a direct relationship between the amount of iron introduced into the cells and the degree of peroxidation. Iron chelators with antioxidents allowed the cells to maintain function. Dr. Bacon is now director of Gastroenterology and Hepatology at St. Louis University.

— Washington, D. C., Walter Reed Army Institute of Research, William H. Crosby, MD, in the Distinguished Physician Program, and colleagues were working to discover the mechanism of iron metabolism. Crosby made a presentation in West Palm Beach, Florida, at IOD's two-day Second Symposium. He explained to an audience of patients and physicians that iron is poisonous and has to be controlled. "It is always escorted through the body. — We don't know how it works. Somehow or other the intestine knows you've been to the blood bank and behaves accordingly.

"This is what I call Crosby's First Law. Metabolism is a complex situation that involves a number of steps. The end product of all these steps is the function of the intestine's normal ability to refrain from absorbing available iron that's not needed.

"If it gets into the body, iron has to be put somewhere — some is stored in ferritin — some in the liver — most iron is stored in the liver — spleen. The amount stored in the marrow is pipeline iron. It's iron that has been taken from cells and is on its way back. After the liver gets loaded up, the body starts putting it away other places; that's the way hemochromatosis comes about." We have become aware that iron also stores disastrously in the brain.

— Rennes, France, Marcel Simon, MD, conducted genetic and family studies. Dr. Simon died in the summer of 1988.

— Kansas City, Kansas, the University of Kansas, Barry S. Skikne, MD, and colleagues, have been developing a simpler, cheaper blood test for iron overload screening.

— New York City, Victor Herbert has developed a new type of ferritin test that is not affected by inflamation. The problem with the serum ferritin test in use is that inflamation will cause the number to spike irrespective of iron. For that reason a confirmatory or backup transferrin saturation is used in conjunction with ferritin. Herbert's new test avoids this confusion since it is not affected by inflammation.

—Stockholm, Sweden, Karolinska Institute, Erik Bjorn-

Rasmussen, MD, with his colleagues made a study of ten subjects with primary hemochromatosis in 1979. Bjorn-Rasmussen delivered a paper at IOD's Second Symposium.

"We measured absorption of body iron, erythrocyte incorporation and determination of reaccumulation time.

"To measure absorption, you give the person radioactive iron by mouth; then you wait two weeks to measure with the body counter or blood sample. From this measurement you can know that a certain amount of this iron is contained in the red blood cells. The rest is contained in other tissues of the body.

"If you have an iron deficiency you have a very high absorption. If stores are normal, you have a normal absorption rate — ten percent down to two percent of food iron. If your stores exceed normal level, you have lower absorption.

"We served standardized meals, hamburgers, mashed potatoes and string beans, and also served it to one hundred normal subjects. We know the normal absorption of this meal. After two weeks we measured the subjects in a body counter. You can see low incorporation of iron in the red blood cells along with high absorption.

"All high iron overloaded subjects had a prolonged period of reaccumulation time — two years to come up again to high levels of reaccumulation. The other subjects reaccumulated very fast — all normal subjects — about two or three months.

"One way or another during the development of a person, iron stores build. Then at a certain level, there's a leveling off and stores are maintained; nothing special happens. Iron absorption. I'd like to repeat what Dr. Crosby said five times yesterday. The body's normal ability to refrain from absorbing iron."

— New York, New York, Albert Einstein College of Medicine, Achilles Demetriou, PhD, and colleagues have demonstrated the first report of long-term survival of liver cells transplanted in laboratory rats. Workers transplanted healthy liver cells into two types of rats with genetic liver function defects. First the researchers injected healthy liver cells into rats unable to form bilirubin, a bile pigment. The transplanted cells survived for three weeks and functioned normally, raising the amount of bilirubin in the rats to near normal levels.

The research group then transplanted healthy liver cells into rats genetically deficient in the protein albumin. Again the cells functioned normally and albumin levels rose.

The ability to transplant liver cells some day may lead to an effective therapy to treat cases of liver failure. Transplanted cells might, for example, take over the function of a liver damaged by toxins such as iron, and allow the injured liver to rest and heal.

— Mayo Clinic, Rochester, Minnesota, doctors are doing liver transplants in humans, including patients with hemochromatosis.

— Australia, University of Queensland, Lawrie Powell, MD, PhD, and colleagues, conduct HLA typing of homozygotes and heterozygotes and twenty year studies of families that made possible the predictive accuracy of transferrin saturation and serum ferritin testing. Mark Bassett, MD, and June Halliday, MD with Powell found that the combination of transferrin saturation above 50 percent and serum ferritin above 200 in men was 94 percent sensitive and that the same saturation with serum ferritin above 150 in women was 86 percent specific for the detection of hemochromatosis in young patients. [Hepatology 1986;6:24-29].

— Joplin, Missouri, William H. Crosby, MD, now retired from Chapman Regional Cancer Center, was conducting studies of patients with hemochromatosis and cancer.

— Hanover, New Hampshire, Walter G. Frey, III, MD, Dartmouth Medical School, has long studied hemochromatosis in the New England population. An Iron Club for a long time was active at Dartmouth. Its members were from a number of medical specialties. This serves to avoid the problem of each blind man describing his own small section of an elephant that Frey often sees. This happens because of the variety of types of specialists working with iron overloaded patients. Frey wrote in the New England Journal of Medicine (256:7-12 July 6 1961) that liver biopsies should be vigorously pursued on relatives of patients. It's the fastest way to uncover those with early, asymptomatic cases. Frey had found that blood tests, transferrin saturation, can be normal in early stages. Even simpler than the biopsy is to begin taking blood, which will rule out or confirm excess iron - **and no harm done.** "Failure to find increased amounts of iron in the bone marrow does not exclude the diagnosis of hemochromatosis." In the same paper Frey said that excess iron deposits in the liver are among the last to be exhausted.

— Dusseldorf, Germany, Claus Niederau, MD, PhD, Georg Strohmeyer, MD and colleagues, University of Dusseldorf, have made extensive studies of the survival rates of treated hemochromatosis patients relative to timeliness of diagnosis and vigor of treatment.

— Worcester, Massachusetts, Herbert Bonkovsky, MD, Director of the Division of Digestive Diseases and Nutrition and of the Center for Study of Disorders of Iron and Porphyrin Metabolism at the Medical Center of the University of Massachusetts and Professor of Medicine, Biochemistry and Molecular Biology, has a long-standing interest in clinical and basic research studies relevant to iron storage disease. Recent work of Dr. Bonkovsky's group has focused on the role of new imaging studies (CT, MRI) for diagnosis and follow-up of hemochromatosis and on the role of iron in production of liver damage and alterations of liver metabolism. He is an expert in porphyria cutanea tarda, as well.

— New York, New York, Victor Herbert, MD JD, Mount Sinai School of Medicine, is investigating nutrient interactions.

North Palm Beach, Florida, IOD has participated in programs at University of Illinois with Richard L. Nelson, MD, to estimate cancer incidence in heterozygotes and at California School of Professional Psychology with Elizabeth Huesman, to study mood swings in males with hemochromatosis, as well as a number of other projects..

IOD has conducted two surveys to determine cost and difficulty in establishing a diagnosis, as well as the race, sex, age and national origins of patients. Conclusions were that all races, both sexes, ages from newborn to one hundred, and those of all national origins, as well as other species are affected.

Much research is going on everywhere in the world. That research, however, doesn't scratch the surface of the kind of research and work and resources that are needed to solve the problems of a secret, silent epidemic.

We are beginning to see the tip of a giant iceberg. "An iceberg's underwater mass is seven times the size of what shows on the surface," says a fictional character in the best-selling novel, "Iceberg," by Clive Cussler.

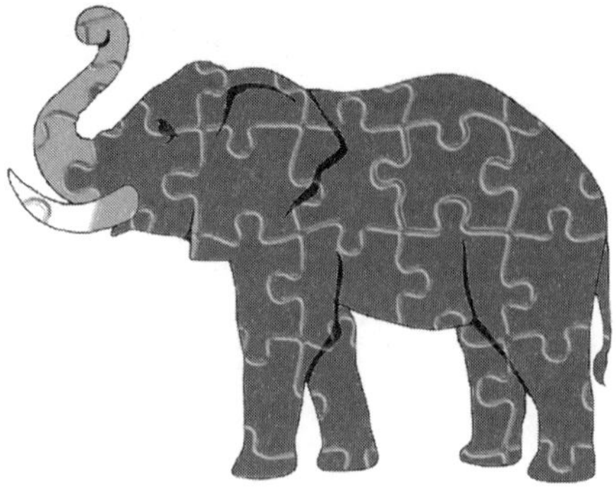

Chapter 19

Research Must Be Stepped Up

A son whose mother's hemochromatosis was diagnosed while she lay dying said bitterly, "She didn't die of hemochromatosis, she died of ignorance."

In my earliest days of research and interviewing scientists, I asked one geneticist, "Since iron is a metal, why couldn't a magnetic device be developed to detect the iron?"

The geneticist gave me a long look and replied, "That is a completely naive idea."

Not many months later I began hearing the first reports of various patients who were setting off airport security alarms. Those patients who knew they were iron overloaded tried to explain the phenomenon to skeptical officials, while undiagnosed patients were as confused as the operators. In some cases, the incidents did lead to belated diagnosis.

Unfortunately airport detectors lack the sensitivity to catch early cases. The detectors are not standardized.

Why couldn't a magnet detect iron? That is precisely what the SQUID is being developed to do. Now, call the idea naive, why could not a magnetic device draw iron from the body? A possibility for the future.

Phlebotomy therapy unloads iron, but is exceedingly slow, requiring months or years. What about blood loss combined with chelation? The ideal chelator would have to be effective, safe, cheap, orally administrated, without unpleasant side effects. An oral chelator is being used in India for thalassemic children, but has not been approved in the U.S. by the FDA. There seems to be still some problems with it. However researchers say Deferiprone is being successfully administered to the 6,000 to 8,000 children born each year in India.

Numerous investigators are working to develop a suitable oral iron-chelating agent.

Better yet, go back to the genes. We must identify the other abnormal mutations to complete the picture. We need to learn how to interfere with the gene, modify it and give it the capability to improve the body's ability to refrain from absorbing too much iron.

Research is needed that would delineate an index, showing an individual's rate of iron absorption, minimum and maximum.

The two most cruel problems of this disease are the lack of prompt diagnosis and the reluctance of physicians to administer vigorous treatment. Physicians and patients are going to have to work together to find the more than a million and a half Americans affected. Most of them can be successfully treated.

A small explosion of discoveries is making the medical community view iron with new eyes. We must give adequate support to the scientists who are dedicated to developing needed information and discovering the missing pieces. Screening programs are essential. New diagnostic tools must be devised. However, I must admit that right now we do have enough information to save almost everyone's life. We just are not doing it.

Diagnosis is not yet perfect. But when there is a question there is one sure way to find out if you do have any excess iron. Start giving blood weekly until you become untreatable by virtue of anemia. Set a cutoff of hematocrit (30 - 35 percent) or hemoglobin (10) and continue the program until you fall below those points. No harm is done and all that happens is that you will unload some excess iron.

Questions were raised at a meeting of the Centers for Disease Control. Some wanted to know: how can we tell if it is really hemochromatosis? Or hemosiderosis? Victor Herbert said, "The question is: is it iron overload?"

Since iron is a toxic poison that everyone has to have, the question should not be: do I have a disease? The question should be: how much iron do I have?

Corwin Q. Edwards, MD, describes the ideal diagnostic test as "one with 100 percent sensitivity, specificity, positive and negative predictive ability, complete safety and widespread availability at modest cost."

Edwards has made a listing of the research areas of iron overload that should be studied. "Research in hemochromatosis will give answers to important questions about normal and abnormal metabolism. Each of the questions posed here needs to be answered.

"1. What are additional mutations? The genetic defect is most likely a defect in the regulation of iron uptake by intestinal mucosal cells. The defective gene product has been largely identified. It may act by failing to give the duodenum a signal to decrease iron absorption even after body iron stores are massively increased; it may prevent the signal from reaching the mucosal cells of the intestine; or it may give a message to the duodenum to continue iron absorption even after iron stores are increased. There are more mutations waiting to be discovered.

"2. What is the frequency of hemochromatosis in the general population? Several groups of investigators are studying this question.

"3. Does a hemochromatosis allele (either one or two) contribute to the iron loading present in some individuals with other disorders?

"If about 12 percent of the general population carries one hemochromatosis gene, about one-eighth of people with any other condition should also be heterozygous for hemochromatosis. There is increasing evidence that individuals who are massively iron loaded and have some other disorder are likely hemochromatosis homozygotes. Evidence is quite good for the presence of one or two HLA-linked hemochromatosis allele to explain iron loading in some individuals who have B-thalassemia minor, hereditary spherocytosis, idiopathic refractory sideroblastic anemia or porphyria cutanea tarda. Systematic study of iron stores in patients who have a disorder associated with increased iron stores should provide insight into the interaction of the hemochromatosis alleles in other conditions.

"4. Will early detection and treatment prevent the complications of hemochromatosis?

"This is a point that has major importance in terms of declining health, decreased productivity and economic loss. It has not yet been proved that all the complications of hemochromatosis are preventable, but it seems reasonable to expect improved health and longevity if affected individuals are identified and treated at a young age. This can be proved by long-term follow-up of a large group of individuals who are found and treated before complications are present."

IOD's experience with many thousands of patients and their physicians over 20 years can almost reply "yes" to that question. In our history the only patients who were diagnosed early enough, before suffering symptoms, have been the relatives of patients. Many of these asymptomatic patients are successfully treated and report to us they feel wonderful

"5. Are transferrin receptors abnormal in people who have hemochromatosis?

"There is a great deal of interest in transferrin receptors at present. Regulation of transferrin receptor number and presumably the regulation of movement of iron from plasma into cells is normal in individuals who are homozygous for hemochromatosis. Movement of iron from one vascular cellular compartment to another will be understood better after transferrin receptor physiology is studied further.

"6. Does hepatic cirrhosis resolve after years of iron depletion therapy?

"Liver disease is one of the worst and commonest complications of hemochromatosis. Some investigators consider cirrhosis to be reversible, while many think it is not improved after phlebotomy therapy. This difference in perception can be resolved by performing repeat liver biopsy after years of vigorous phlebotomy therapy in patients whose initial biopsy revealed cirrhosis."

IOD has learned that timid treatment does not work. The patient's goal is to prevent liver cancer, which occurs too often even after all iron is cleaned out. You reach your goal by being vigorous in treatment and taking ferritin far below what labs are saying is normal. Give the liver a chance to repair itself.

"7. Is the hypogonadism in hemochromatosis usually secondary (pituitary damage) or tertiary (hypothalmic damage)?

"It is clear that direct testicular damage (primary hypogonadism) is not the usual cause of hypogonadism in patients with hemochromatosis. Inadequate information exists in the literature about distinction of secondary from possible tertiary hypogonadism. Repeated administration of clomiphene (by mouth) or LHRH (parenterally) followed by measurement of LH, FSH, testosterone, dihydrotesterone, and determination of response to repeat LHRH stimulation in individuals with at least secondary hypogonadism should provide important information about iron damage to pituitary and hypothalamus."

In the future when we fully understand how the mutations operate, that's when we can prevent its effect. We might educate the gene, retrain the gene to send its products to the point of entry to stand guard at the iron gate.

IOD now recommends that we can forget "diagnosis." Find high iron. Lower it. "When to do the screening has an easy answer," wrote G. J Escobar, MD. "That is, as soon as you think about it." So think about it.

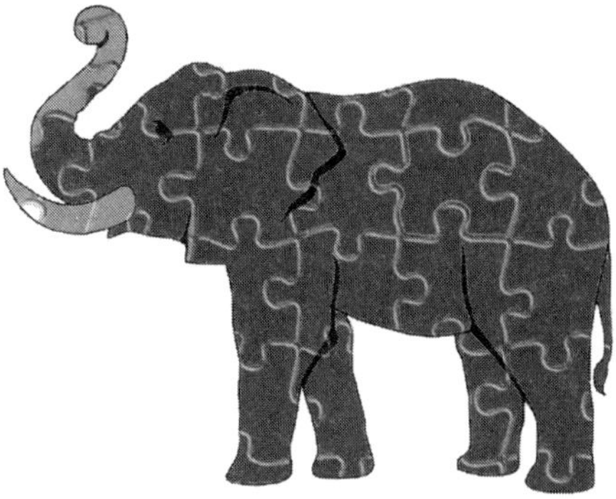

Part 8

"Can it be prevented?"

Chapter 20

The Sacrificial Sibling

A twenty-nine-year-old Jacksonville, Florida woman died in January, 1990. An autopsy revealed hemochromatosis. "Since the disease was so rare," wrote a sister, the rest of the family never had the testing." Their brother began suffering symptoms similar to those of his sister, and he received a diagnosis of diabetes in October, 1991. Too late, he was found to be iron overloaded. He died on Christmas Eve. He was twenty-seven.

If you are related to an individual who has received a correct diagnosis of iron overload, you should have the best hope of receiving a pre-injury diagnosis. With the present low priorities that are being assigned to iron tests, relatives have a much better chance of avoiding damage than the general public. Relatives are more likely than others to get early discovery and removal of excess iron. The first patient in the family — the Sacrificial Sibling — is the one most likely to suffer needless disability or death until iron tests become routine.

"The early diagnosis of hemochromatosis, at a time when it can be treated effectively," says Virgil F. Fairbanks, MD, "will continue to be elusive until physicians routinely rcquest assay of SI and

TIBC, or serum ferritin, as part of a general medical examination."

Physicians are beginning to request these tests, and laboratories have started including them in their routine blood work.

Marilyn, a registered nurse in Chicago, received a diagnosis while she is still able to work, not, however, before the iron caused injury. Marilyn had watched her brother die only two months earlier. His diagnosis was made just before death. Marilyn said she feels a responsibility to her family to make sure all blood relatives are tested and that any who are diagnosed are then properly treated.

It isn't always easy to convince relatives.

"It's great for the doctor to be able to identify someone in the family who will serve as master sergeant for the family," said Walter G. Frey, III, MD, at IOD's Second Symposium. "The way I determine that is where the family goes for Thanksgiving. You don't end up with the black sheep. If you're dealing with the black sheep, no one else in the family wants to hear anything he has to say."

— Russell of Hanover, Pennsylvania, was diagnosed after his younger brother died of the disease.

— Benjamin of Middletown, Ohio, was diagnosed along with four brothers and two sisters. Another brother had been treated for diabetes for years. Doctors had not been able to control it. Still, iron was not thought of until it was discovered in his brothers and sisters.

— Bud of Pittsburgh, Pennsylvania, received a diagnosis during a family check after his father was diagnosed. Some family members had been diagnosed with sideroblastic anemia. Authorities suggest that this genetic anemia may remain unexpressed unless it occurs in association with the hemochromatosis gene.

— Joyce of British Columbia is gravely concerned about her twenty-five-year-old son, who is overloaded with iron, his doctor said. Her other son died at twenty-four of "unexplained causes." He had early cirrhosis and other problems. However, "one day he was fine (except tired); the next morning he was dead."

— Pete of San Bernardino, California, was diagnosed, not through family screening, however, although his brother was a patient. The iron was found during surgery.

— Patricia of Wauconda, Illinois, was finally diagnosed, but not until a year after the death of her brother, and thirty years after the death of their father. Patricia had to be persistent with four doctors to get her diagnosis.

— Jane of Gainesville, Florida, said "It comes as a shock that being a good detective, plus a lot of good luck ... can spell the difference between health and illness for yourself and those you care about ..." Her father died of hemochromatosis after spending "years, a fortune and much suffering." His doctor was a prominent physician, but he did not suspect iron.

— Jo Ann of Franklin, Indiana, and her three children all received diagnoses.

"The prevalence of the hemochromatosis allele in many populations is astonishing," wrote Fairbanks in *Hematology 1981* "The full significance of the high gene frequency ... remains to be determined. Interactions between the hemochromatosis allele and other factors appear to be involved in the pathogenesis of idiopathic refractory sideroblastic anemia and of porphyria cutanea tarda.

"The possible adverse effect of iron fortification on food on both heterozygotes and homozygotes requires careful re-examination, especially in view of the unexpectedly high prevalence of carriers ..."

— Mrs. B of Burbank, Ohio, has completed two years of weekly phlebotomies for hemochromatosis, and is now on a maintenance schedule of four treatments a year. Her aunt had died of cirrhosis of the liver. Doctors at the clinic suspect the aunt died of undiagnosed hemochromatosis.

— Peggy of Elko, Nevada, knows about hemochromatosis, which is being treated in her husband and two children.

— Dudley of Georgetown, Louisiana, his brother and his son are all being treated. Dudley's mother had died of "a liver ailment."

— Mary of Sacramento, California, and her sister are both patients.

— Joan of Ukiah, California, had traveled to Mayo Clinic seven years before she received a diagnosis elsewhere following her brother's diagnosis. Now four of eight siblings are identified. At Mayo Joan insisted that "there is something wrong." But she says, "there was no finding." The clinic that diagnosed her first brother had observed his iron level soar for three years, she says, and after the diagnosis doctors failed to tell Dick that his relatives needed to be checked. Their mother had died at age fifty-two of cirrhosis and heart disease. Their mother's mother had also died at fifty-two.

— Laura of Tracytown, Washington, was diagnosed along with two brothers.

— Linda of Guin, Alabama, lost her brother, Ted, in 1972. He had suffered a variety of health problems and his color gradually changed. "He looked like someone with a great tan." The family did not realize his body was like that all over. In the closing weeks of his life, Ted was admitted to a North Florida hospital, where he remained for about two weeks without improvement. His dad got him released and took him to a veterans hospital, where the diagnosis was made. It was too late. Ted died two weeks later. Despite the diagnosis, cause of death was listed as idiopathic myocardiopathy with myocardial insufficiency. (Hemochromatosis is covered up by the diseases it causes.) Ted was thirty-four.

Ted's brother, Paul, died thirteen years later. His autopsy report said that Paul died as a result of severe congestive heart failure due to hemochromatosis. The report said that family screening was mandatory since the "complications of the disorder are potentially preventable by regular phlebotomy." Some medical examiners may be reluctant to "scold" the physician by naming as a cause of death a condition so readily treatable.

Their father died a few months later after numerous blood transfusions for hemolytic anemia. His autopsy report also listed hemochromatosis.

The family's mother had received a diagnosis of "unexplained" cirrhosis of the liver. A determination of hemochromatosis was also added to her diagnosis, but her disease is apparently not as severe as her children's and husband's. A thirty-seven-year-old son was diagnosed during family screening, was treated and is doing well. Another brother was diagnosed, but said he felt all right, didn't believe in doctors, and he rejected treatment. A sister was diagnosed and is being treated.

Betty, the eldest sister, was told by her doctor that her high normal iron levels are of no concern. She has eight children, and has been a regular blood donor for fifteen years. All children of homozygous parents are themselves homozygous for the disease.

— John of Long Valley, New Jersey, received an early diagnosis after his mother died, diagnosed too late. He says his mother's correct diagnosis gave him "the gift of life." John's wife is a nurse and "had never heard of" iron overload. "I could find absolutely no information in any of my nursing books," she said.

— Alice of Hamilton, Illinois, is receiving treatment, but her older brother died in August, 1985.

— Charles of Riverside, Connecticut, was treated for twenty-nine years for arthritis and other problems before his recent diagnosis. His father had died young, and his uncle had had "heart problems."

— Roxanne of Tucson, Arizona, was waiting along with her doctors before undergoing a liver biopsy, after showing high iron levels "for at least ten years" and then developing abnormal liver enzymes. While waiting, though, her son called her from another city. He too had received a report of abnormal liver function.

— Jeanne of Morrisville, Pennsylvania, was diagnosed after losing her sister to the disease.

— June of Milwaukee, Wisconsin, was diagnosed after great difficulty, but her diagnosis did lead to that of her sister.

— Richard of White River Junction, Vermont, and a sister were diagnosed.

— Wendy of Wisconsin was diagnosed along with two daughters.

— Joe of California was diagnosed with two brothers, but a sister died at thirty-eight.

On Nov. 14, 1985, the New England Journal of Medicine published a report of a study in Dusseldorf, Germany, that detailed the "Survival and causes of death in cirrhotic and in noncirrhotic patients with primary hemochromatosis." Claus Niederau, MD, PhD, and his colleagues had analyzed the causes of death of one hundred sixty-three patients from 1959 to 1983. The study shows that life expectancy is reduced in patients whose excess iron is not found until after the event of cirrhosis, compared with earlier diagnoses. The same is true of patients who have already developed diabetes, compared with those who are diagnosed in earlier stages.

Life expectancy was also reduced in patients whose iron burden was too great to be removed within eighteen months, compared with those who could be de-ironed in that time.

The study showed that liver cancer was 219 times more frequent among hemochromatosis patients; that enlarged heart was 306 times more frequent; liver cirrhosis was 13 times more frequent and diabetes was seven times more frequent than among the general population. Seven of the patients died from cancer other than liver cancer.

What caused such a stir in the scientific community was the evidence that patients who were diagnosed before the onset of cirrhosis and had their iron removed within eighteen months could expect a normal life span.

Niederau concluded the paper by saying that "The present study demonstrates that early diagnosis in the noncirrhotic stage of hemochromatosis can improve the patient's prognosis to normal life expectancy and may also prevent the late development of liver cancer. These findings therefore encourage programs of screening for this disease, which is still often underdiagnosed or diagnosed too late."

David L. Witte, MD PhD, says "Could we not do better?"

Workers at University of Rochester (New York) School of Medicine conducted a study in 1990 on the cost-effectiveness of screening the population for hemochromatosis.

"Not cost-effective" has been the most often used argument against screening.

Pradyumna D. Phatak, MD, and colleagues constructed a "decision tree." The variables they used were (1) prevalence (2) probability of developing symptoms (3) cost of the test (4) discount rate for quantity testing.

Researchers found there was a net benefit from screening in the "most plausible case," which presumes a prevalence of three per thousand, a test cost of $12, a fifty percent chance of developing symptoms and a discount rate of three percent. The doctors concluded that screening is indeed cost-effective.

Is it cost-effective to save a life? To save a whole family?

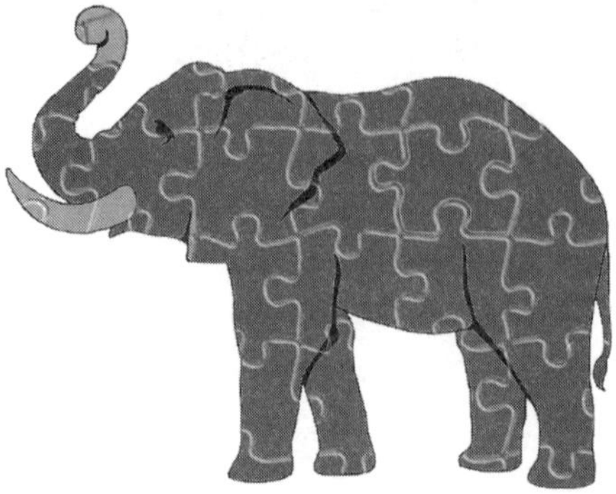

Chapter 21

The Cost: Malpractice, Fortunes, Lives

The first malpractice case of missed diagnosis and delayed treatment of hemochromatosis was filed in 1985 in New Jersey. The case was settled out of court for half a million dollars. It was the experience of a man who had suffered vague symptoms as early as 1968. Except for his sister's diagnosis, he probably would have died undiagnosed. Brother and sister exchanged notes, and it was she who first realized that what John had was hemochromatosis.

John and his wife, Hedwig, had spent large sums on futile medical bills over years of misdiagnosis. In addition to the medical bills was the cost of lost income, as John's illness continued to advance.

John says his first symptom was "being washed out and tired all the time." It was a slow, insidious thing. In 1968 John left his job in Cleveland and returned to his home in New Jersey. He was working as Quotation Manager for a firm that was part of Harvard Industries.

No matter what he did, John could not shake the fatigue. In 1972 a new symptom appeared in the form of a black stool that indicated internal bleeding. John was taken to an emergency room. At that time a liver biopsy was performed, and it revealed cirrhosis. The biopsy also revealed excessive iron. A physician involved said that John needed to be bled, and that his family should be notified to be tested. However other medical opinions were that John's condition ruled out phlebotomies, so the iron was ignored.

Arthritis gradually entered the picture, but John said, "You sort of get used to it."

In 1978 came an attack of angina pectoris. John still had not heard the word, hemochromatosis, and still had no knowledge that it was the iron causing his problems. By now John and Hedwig had moved to a new town and a new physician. John asked his new doctor, "Why am I so tired all the time?" The answer was that the angina was doing it. A coronary by-pass was advised. John decided to submit to the operation. Afterwards, though, he was disappointed that the by-pass did nothing to help the fatigue.

John's sister, Alice, lived not too far away. She began experiencing some of the same symptoms as John's. Her tests showed an enlarged liver. Of course doctors kept questioning her about her drinking habits, the amount of her alcoholic intake. Her family knew better than that! Alcohol was not the problem. Doctors were going to have to find another cause of the liver damage. Luckily for Alice — and for John — her diagnosis of hemochromatosis was made in 1981. She began immediate treatment.

The day Alice had her first phlebotomy, John and Hedwig were visiting. John and Alice started talking. They compared their bronze skin, red palms, and other symptoms.

"You know what I think, John? ..."

"Yes."

"John, go get tested."

John's tests did reveal hemochromatosis. Meanwhile, though, he had developed diabetes to add to his other troubles.

It was hard for John to realize that out of the number of doctors he had consulted, none of them could recognize this disease. He wondered how much his life had been shortened by this ignorance. He wondered how he would be able to provide for his wife. The monetary award will help to answer that. As for his own life, well, John tried to keep working. He still required lots of sleep. He just did the best he could until he died February 14, 1990.

John decided to accept an out-of-court settlement, and says the case was finally settled on the courthouse steps. Medicare and other insurance plans have been slow to cover the small cost of treatment. We have written to those agencies, telling them that they are already covering many clients who are undiagnosed. As a result such people will cost them big time down the road. I call it Insurance Insanity.

-William of Gloucester City New Jersey is amazed that Medicare declined a nominal payment at a blood bank, but is willing to pay $762.28 each time at a hospital.

-Richard of Springfield Ohio is distressed that his primary care physician's lab has stopped including iron screens in routine testing. Richard said that the insurance companies forced the change. Talk about shooting yourself in the foot.

-Bob of Lakewood Colorado is puzzled by the lack of interest shown by the media. Speaking of the *60 MINUTES* fiasco he remembers a "firestorm" surrounding Alar and apples. He says, "Probably not even one death can be attributed to Alar. Yet here are more than a million unsuspecting Americans being pushed toward their graves by their supposedly healthy breakfast cereals." I call these breakfasts "cereal killers."

Hemochromatosis is the cheapest of diseases, both to detect and to treat *..unless it's neglected.* When neglected, we have heard of every kind of horror story. A South Carolina woman was "miserable for two years" before diagnosis, despite her brother's diagnosis. Now she is being treated, and has given eight gallons of blood. There is no reason that her blood cannot be used. But she says "the expense is terrific." She had to sell her home.

This woman's mother asks, "Why can't iron levels be tested along with all the other blood tests they do during a physical?"

Ray Yip MD, formerly of the Centers for Disease Control agrees. "Iron testing will give you a higher yield on results," he says, "something you can do something about, than other tests that are now standard." Cost effective!

-Bill in Florida was seeing a hematologist for three years. His saturation was 92 percent and his ferritin was 1200. He was being treated for arthritis. When he heard about IOD Bill wanted to be tested for iron. His physician turned him over to a gastroenterologist with a sneering request "to appease the patient, do a CT and liver biopsy, because, though he shows no indications of hemochromatosis, he wants to rule it out." During those three years Bill could have been de-ironed! We'd like to hold this doctor up as a horrible example, but he's just typical. Bill had to struggle to receive a correct diagnosis.

We don't want to do any doctor bashing. Too many great physicians help us in our membership. When reporting facts, these are the kinds of facts we receive to report.

— Anna in Kentucky said, "I cannot find a doctor to sit down and discuss this with me. My family doctor says he never had a case before (twenty-five years in practice) and says he is learning about it from me. ... I am happy they can use my blood or I would feel even worse." Anna's brother had "high iron tests" but was only instructed to give blood twice a year.

And from others: "I have been told by one doctor I had this and by another I didn't need to give blood to help."

— Elsewhere: "Her doctor told her that she had an overabundance of red blood cells, and warned her to discontinue taking vitamin tablets containing iron, to limit red meats to once weekly, not eat beans, but that she could eat fish. Since this limits her food intake drastically ... we are at a loss."

Americans are in the grip of unmanageable medical costs that drain insurance funds. The neglect of a common and treatable disease is costing our nation's people enormously in misspent money for medical bills. The neglect costs us even more in destroyed health and shortened lives.

David Witte MD PhD, speaking at IOD's 15th Annual Symposium said, "Primarily in our country we have a disease care system instead of a health care system." At his lab in Ottumwa Iowa workers perform UIBC (unsaturated iron binding capacity) for two cents each, which will point the way to further testing. Witte says, "Add serum iron for another nickel. Add TIBC and we're up to a dime."

Lloyd H Smith Jr MD, Associate Dean at University of California, San Francisco, said, "The diagnosis is more frequently missed than made." Certainly an understatement. You can see why the word "incredible" crops up so often.

Here are a few more comments that come in daily from patients. "They obviously never thought to check his iron levels ... it's almost unbelievable." (Marianne in Sudbury Massachusetts, after her husband received two heart transplants).

"I am a 34-year-old RN. It took me only five years to get diagnosed! (SfosterRN1 on the Internet).

"The dog food manufacturers arc doing more harm than automobiles." (John in York, Pennsylvania, a fancier of Dalmatians).

"It took four years to diagnose. I was almost suicidal." (Marvin in Texas).

An Indiana woman's brother did commit suicide.

"Your symptoms aren't right for hemochromatosis. Come back in a year," was told to Lois in New Jersy. Her ferritin was 1290.

"How tragic that I could someday be sending you a memorial for my sons because I could not explain the urgency .. And their uninformed doctors would not take the information seriously." (Katherine in Mississippi).

"I'm damn mad that this is such a secret." (Mary in Lancaster California).

"My doctor doesn't believe women my age can have it." (Cathy of Riverside, California).

Enough! But those reports keep rolling in on our poor telephones and in our mail every hour. A doctor on the Internet said, "It's time for patients to stop being intimidated by ill-informed and poorly trained physicians. I know it's tough," he said, "but people have to stand up for their medical rights." It is the patient's life and the patient's death.

The current American infatuation with iron is dangerous!

In view of the malpractice crisis in the United States, it is not good news to report that many more cases will be filed, will be settled in court or out, and many more awards will be made because of injury to patients resulting from medical ignorance of iron overload. These litigations reflect the frustration of families who discover that their loss was caused by medical lack of awareness.

A second malpractice case was settled out of court in March, 1987, this time against the U. S. government.

The United States District Court for the District of Colorado stipulated in a compromise settlement, "The defendant, United States of America, will pay the sum of $75,000 to George and Margot Singer." In addition to the lump amount, George was awarded disability payment of $18,000 per year plus medical care estimated to be a quarter of a million dollars, because of his widespread body damage.

George was disabled at age thirty-four.

He received his belated diagnosis of hemochromatosis in June, 1984. "I was very ill," he says, "and emotionally stressed" when a hematologist said his prognosis was extremely poor with hepatic and/or cardiac failure almost certain.

Even with treatment, George was told, he could expect to live about two years.

Five years after that dreadful prognosis, George was still alive, still prevailing over his many problems of arthritis, cirrhosis, diabetes, esophageal varices, impotence, ascites, osteoporosis, chronic diarrhea and heart disease.

George had served in the U. S. Army until his medical retirement for physical disability in August, 1978. Arthritis was the disability. Hemochromatosis could have been diagnosed at that time. Or the diagnosis should have been made even earlier, in 1968, when George first underwent examination for arthritis symptoms.

The medical care provided by the Army and later continued by the Veterans Administration, was deficient.

The Army had also ignored other evidence of hemochromatosis. While this medical misfeasance was going on, George developed more serious consequences: liver dysfunction that progressed to cirrhosis; arthritis that continued to become more severe and widespread; diabetes; heart disease and incapacitating fatigue. The fatigue along with the other problems became so intractable that George had to give up his livelihood.

Medical testimony in the case recorded that George's "career and quality of life have been destroyed by this formidable disease, that with competent medical service, should have been recognized, diagnosed and treated well before most of these irreversible complications occurred."

The case did not go to trial. George had rejected previously a much more generous settlement offer from the government. His attorney, James S. Bertagnolli, said he is "very unhappy with the way the government handled the case," stalling, spending perhaps $50,000 fighting it. For George to take it to court, would have cost him an additional $10,000 to $12,000, he said.

The government's stalling did work to its advantage as George became weary with it, and to cap it off, he and his wife ran into bad luck on an Indiana highway during a visit to his family. A car smashed into theirs and injured them both seriously. The accident demolished George's morale. He gave up the fight.

The government fought the case with its big guns. They spent huge sums and they were able to find doctors who testified that an early diagnosis would not have changed the course of George's disease; they claimed that "there is little evidence of dramatic improvement following phlebotomy in hemochromatosis."

This is not true.

But remember ... that word, hemochromatosis. Doctors are accustomed to seeing "hemochromatosis" patients in late stages, possibly too late for effective treatment.

There is now abundant evidence for doctors who keep themselves updated, that phlebotomy treatment does indeed result in improvement and in fact that phlebotomy therapy can save the life of the patient, if instituted early and vigorously.

Did George win? You may be asking how $75,000 and the other benefits are going to make up for the injury that has been done to him. Of course it can't.

George would like to turn back the calendar. He would like to be whisked back in time to those days in the Army when his symptoms first appeared. Knowing what he knows now, he wishes he could go back and get the correct diagnosis and proper treatment to restore his health and give him the years of life he will now miss.

George's main concern now is to "gain attention from the medical profession." He hopes the fact of the award will "help physicians to suspect iron overload in their patients."

If you think hemochromatosis was finished with George, it was not. It had to break his heart by killing his sister, Lula, 39, and his brother, John, 44. He has another brother, who is seriously affected. Finally — at last — a member of the family has received an early diagnosis, Martha, George's sister in Peru, Indiana. Her excess iron was detected before any damage. Martha's iron is now being speedily unloaded. (An example in the plaintiff's own family that phlebotomy treatment does result in improvement, and even in the prevention of damage).

Nearly 100 million of the U.S. population - now 270,000,000-

suffer from chronic ailments. Three-fourths of the nation's medical expense goes for heart disease, arthritis, cancer, diabetes, ulcers and AIDs, which includes orthopedic replacement and organ transplants, but does not include home nursing care. The cost exceeds $230 billion a year.

Is that enough money to care about? The cost of treating those diseases is killing America's health care system. Putting it all together, iron is a high-priced player in the system. The neglect of iron overload creates great holes in the system that allows billions of dollars to flow through without good result.

The insurance industry endures heavy and unnecessary financial losses because of medical negligence of iron overload. Ironically enough, patients who are struggling with hemochromatosis, undiagnosed or misdiagnosed as some other condition, have less trouble finding insurance than those patients who are accurately diagnosed and are under treatment. Thomas of Orlando was actually diagnosed as a result of an insurance exam that required testing for iron. After his diagnosis, though, "the company decided they wanted no part of me and would not consider issuance of any life coverage," Tom wrote.

Meanwhile that company should think about this. The company has without knowing it re-imbursed large amounts for claims to their insured parties who have not enjoyed the benefit of early diagnosis. Prevention has to be cheaper for all concerned.

Health insurers and employers have already paid out millions in avoidable (and futile) medical bills. Individuals have spent fortunes in pursuit of a correct diagnosis. Those who cannot afford high-priced care are suffering for lack of medical care; those who can afford the very best care are suffering from the quality of the care.

Projecting the IOD Survey revelation of medical costs misspent in search of a correct diagnosis of hemochromatosis, onto the U. S. population, health insurers, employers and individuals should prepare for the following medical expenses (unless awareness increases sufficiently):

— ten percent of America's one point five million gene carriers for hemochromatosis — 150,000 people — will spend an average each of more than $5,000, (1984 dollars), or a total of over half a billion wasted dollars.

— four percent will spend "fortunes" and end in financial ruin.

— twenty-two percent will spend "unknown" amounts, all in pursuit of a correct diagnosis.

These last two groups can't be calculated and therefore can't be projected numerically.

Put all these doomed people together in a stadium and announce that without proper care they are each and every one dying, and what would happen? The outcry would be heard to the moon. CNN would send coverage. The media would swarm. Talk shows would be shrieking.

But these are not gathered in a mob, they are not identified. They don't know they are dying. So there is no outcry. Certain segments of society depend on this misspent money. Victor Herbert, speaking of the tobacco industry and of the vitamin C industry, calls it "murder for money."

Someone has said our new century will be different, better. Let's pray it is.

In another hundred years people will discuss our present-day medical practices and describe them as horrifying. Someone is going to write a historical piece like the following:

"Twentieth Century doctors became so influential and sought after that most of them took on many more patients than they could properly treat. Patients, no matter how ill, were required to make the trip to the doctors, whether in their offices or in hospitals. Many doctors ran patients through their examining rooms, as on a conveyer belt, devoting about ten minutes to each. Standard treatment consisted of the writing of a prescription for drugs. Sometimes the drugs helped, but often they only added to the patient's misery. Iron was one of the most popular prescriptions.

"Doctors were just beginning to learn of the fatal consequences of excess iron toward the end of the century. It has been suggested that present day iron detectors, if passed over an old cemetery, would raise a horrendous racket."

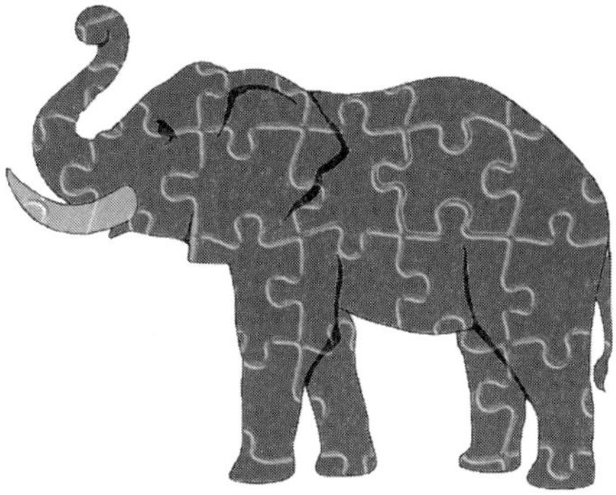

Chapter 22

Look At Iron With New Eyes

The iron elephant is beginning to come together, but stray left-over parts dangle. More work is needed to put the creature into clear focus. Conflicting views of experts have been presented here, as well as perceptions not in agreement with the text. Many authorities will disagree with portions of this book, just as they disagree with one another. IOD feels confident that we have learned what works and what does not because iron overload has been our exclusive mission day and night for twenty years. As the pieces of this elephant line up, we have to be willing to recognize changes with wide open eyes and wide open minds.

Forget the rusty "information" that tired means "iron poor blood." Forget the idea that you have to work and scheme to get enough iron into your diet. Consider yourself lucky if your metabolism is in normal working order and has the ability to turn away excess iron.

Recognize that iron is abundant in foods, and though not all iron is available for absorption, that fact just gives your rejecting mechanism less work. Know that unless you are losing blood, you can get rid of only one milligram of iron per day in body detritus, shed cells. Ask yourself why the recommended daily intake (RDI) for iron was set at fifteen milligrams for adult women as late as 1990. Stop worrying about a little spilled blood. Tell yourself you are relieving iron stores. Donate at the blood bank! See iron in a new light!

Don't ignore early symptoms. Some of the same symptoms associated with anemia can also be the result of iron overload. Fatigue is one of the earliest. You may find you require more sleep. At work you may find yourself counting the hours before your head can find a pillow. With some kinds of chronic fatigue, you don't realize how tired you actually were, until you start feeling better.

Don't tell yourself you're "getting old." Chronic fatigue is not natural.

Joint pain, especially in the hands, should be investigated. Don't let a doctor start treating the pain without checking iron levels.

Lessening libido. All in the mind? Psychological? Maybe not. Check iron levels.

Long before abnormal liver function tests show the abnormality, your liver struggles to do its work. Abdominal cramping and bouts of diarrhea can be symptoms of iron overload.

However, if your objective is to prevent body injury, don't wait for symptoms. Know what your iron levels are. Keep your medical records in your own file. You paid for them. You care more about them than any medical group. Learn what they mean. If your doctor won't give you copies of your own records, find one who will.

Don't take iron. Now that you are looking at iron with new eyes, you will not be medicating with iron when you are tired and rundown. You will not allow iron to be included with vitamins in the belief that iron can't hurt.

You're an athlete? A long distance runner? All the more reason to avoid iron supplements. You are working for body strength, not body breakdown. Do you want to spend money for expensive feces? Nutritionists say that when you buy and ingest excessive amounts of nutrients the body can't use, you are creating expensive urine. In the case of iron, you can't count on that's being the only damage. You can only hope.

Don't allow your doctor to give you iron. Ah! So now you know more than your doctor, do you? About iron, maybe yes, if iron is prescribed simply on the basis of low red cell counts.

Insist that your physician dig deeper and find the true cause of low counts and other signs.

Routine iron following surgery? Not you!

There are enough American women to populate an entire state who have had iron wrongly prescribed. Those who were able to refrain from absorbing it, suffered pain only in their checkbooks. For others it was a deadly prescription.

A woman in Yonkers, New York, was given Trinsicon for years. Now she is having to bleed to unload that excess iron. She paid for it going in and is paying for it going out.

Tom in Utah is a beneficiary of early detection, he says, and he feels truly fortunate that he was in a blood bank donating blood and became part of the university screening program. He was told that having been a blood donor all his adult life had worked to his advantage. Now at fifty-one he feels well and optimistic about prospects for a normal life.

Read the labels. Be logical. Why would you want 100 percent of your day's "requirement" for iron in your breakfast cereal? Food processors gain an advertising and commercial advantage by adding iron to packaged, canned and frozen foods. You don't have to be a mathematician to recognize that you can't avoid iron. People who eat foods in their natural state will receive enough iron to maintain a balance and must hope their rejecting mechanism is working to turn away the excess.

When transfusions are necessary, protect yourself during long-term transfusion therapy. A chelation drug is supportive. Desferal, the best known, can be infused by pump. The same protection is needed by patients on hemodialysis. The blood cleansing procedure leads to iron overload. When these patients become anemic, too many physicians prescribe iron, unaware that hemodialysis is an iron loading condition!

Pressure the Food and Nutrition Board to lower iron's RDI. If an RDI is to have any practical value, it should be an accurate reflection of the human body's requirement. Keeping in mind individual variations, it is difficult enough to set standards for any nutrient. But iron is a one-way nutrient with no outlet, a toxic cancer-causing substance in excess that needs particular discretion.

The RDIs for iron are currently set at ten milligrams for infants six months to ten years; children ten to seventeen are advised by the Food and Nutrition Board to consume an additional two milligrams for males and five for females.

The former sixty milligrams for pregnant and lactating women was lowered in 1989 to fifteen milligrams during pregnancy and no supplements recommended during lactation. With the increase in reported neonatal hemochromatosis and iron overload in not-yet-born babies, even these levels deserve re-examination.

Victor Herbert, MD, JD, authored the report, "The Recommended Dietary Allowance (RDA) for Iron Proposed by the 1980-1985 Tenth Committee on Dietary Allowances Impaneled by the National Academy of Sciences," published in the American Journal of Clinical Nutrition in 1987 as the RDI for iron, and edited and published in 1989 as the 10th RDA by the Academy. Note: RDA has been changed to RDI.

Herbert is professor of medicine at Mount Sinai School of Medicine in New York and is Chief of Hematology and Nutrition Laboratory at Bronx VA Medical Center.

The report noted that absorption increases as iron stores become depleted and decreases as stores increase. "This fact probably explains the lower-than-expected incidence of iron deficiency among people consuming diets containing less than the RDA for iron ..."

The average American woman may be consuming only two-thirds of her "daily needs," as stipulated by the inflated recommended daily allowances. Why then, is she not iron deficient? "Most women are not anemic," says Teresa Wright, MD, medical instructor at the University of California San Francisco Medical School, as quoted in SAVVY July, 1986. In the same article, Janet MacDonald, a nutritionist at the FDA, was quoted as saying that some people consume far less iron than the RDA but show "no evidence of iron deficiency,"

Herbert's report says that "one and a half milligram of absorbed iron would meet the RDA for adult women ..."

The committee's recommendations include:

— ten milligrams per day for adult males and postmenopausal women, if the average absorption of food iron is ten percent. By absorbing only ten percent of the iron available in food, the ten milligrams of food iron would more than supply the daily loss of one milligram.

— fifteen milligrams per day for women of child-bearing age, to meet the additional needs imposed by menstrual losses.

Herbert wrote, "There is little direct evidence of a high prevalence of iron deficiency in the elderly. Survey data suggest inflammatory disease, rather than iron deficiency, as the main cause of anemia in the elderly."

A family practitioner at a medical meeting in 1986 in Washington, D.C., shook his head, saying that dosing with iron in nursing homes is a common and dangerous practice.

If the FDA's eyes can't view iron in a realistic light, yours can. As one whose eyes have been opened in a harsh way, I formulate my own RDI for iron, one milligram of assimilable iron to make up daily loss, hoping for the ability to reject all above that, or compensating for the extra intake by maintenance phlebotomies.

"Iron deficiency continues to be overplayed as a public health threat, and hemochromatosis — a real killer — is played down," said William H. Crosby, MD *Nutrition Today, July/August 1986].*

Food companies gain a tremendous advertising advantage by adding iron to their products because of public perception that more iron means more health. Iron holds a seductive position in the public's perception of nutrition. But iron is the most insidious of food additives. The mineral is naturally plentiful in food. Patients who have been lucky enough to be correctly diagnosed, have to make a serious search to find cereals, breads, canned, packaged or frozen foods without iron additives.

Iron deficiency is simple to treat. But should treatment be left to food companies? Who is going to investigate for the cause of the deficiency? Who will look for the cancer, the internal bleeding, the chronic infection?

Crosby has worked to protect the public from excessive iron. "The addition of iron to food is illegal," he says in the above article. While iron is present in many foods, it is well known as a carcinogen in excess. The Delaney Amendment of the Food and Drug and Cosmetic Act prohibits the use of any additives which under any conditions induce cancer in any strain of test animal. The animal suffering highest incidence of iron-caused cancer is the human animal.

"Under 21 USCS & 348(c) Secretary has no discretion to balance beneficial effects of food additive against its danger as carcinogen and may not use his enforcement discretion to authorize continued use of such additive during gradual phase-out period, although he does have discretion to adopt reasonable timetable and procedure to assure orderly removal of such additive from commerce..."

IOD has made presentations to the FDA and to the Orphan Products Board. We told them that an estimated more than one million Americans are genetically and unknowingly absorbing dangerous amounts of iron from an ordinary diet. We told them that the rapidly increasing number of diagnosed cases supports the scientific estimates of the high prevalence of the H gene. We told them that most affected individuals are still unaware that they are absorbing and storing lethal amounts of iron. We told them that iron overload is: deadly ... common ... underdiagnosed ... treatable.

My personal preference of a way to solve the problem of the ubiquitous adding of iron to processed food would be to educate the public about the danger. That would be preferable to passing new laws. Let the public learn, let the public look at iron with new eyes, let the public decide whether it wants to continue buying these products. Let the public read labels. When the public sees iron listed among additives, let the public return the package to the shelf.

Support research. Help awareness. Such awareness will mark a new era in human health. Resistance, caused by ingrained misinformation, is hard to dislodge.

In the Middle Ages Cistercian monks were required to be bled four times a year to tranquilize the body. It wouldn't hurt everybody to follow their example.

Trousseau, a French physician, first described a patient with hemochromatosis in 1865. More than a hundred years ago the disease was recognized as a medical entity. However, diagnosis was made only at autopsy and the disease was thought to be untreatable. Since the pioneering work in 1947 of Drs. Davis and Arrowsmith, medicine has had no excuse for ignoring iron overload diseases.

You yourself may not be a hemochromatosis patient. But someone you know, someone in your family, someone at your place of work, someone, is storing damaging amounts of excess iron. I hope with all my heart that that person has been made aware of the condition and is acting to remove the iron. You may be the one to make a critical difference by helping to create awareness.

Don't think of this as a separate "disease." It is not: do you have "it" or not have "it." Everyone has iron. The only question is how much do you have? If ferritin is well above ten, you'd be wise to become a blood donor and unload the excess. It will only help.

There is no reason for anyone to medicate with iron, unless intestines have been surgically removed or unless the individual can't eat food.

The thirteen percent of the population who carry the single gene, and everybody else for that matter, should use caution, should avoid vitamin C additives or excessive alcohol. What a simple way to preserve your body and extend your life span.

Without question on our planet where all things are possible, we can overcome the crisis of knowledge lack. If necessary we can train ourselves to see old things in a new light. We can look at iron with new eyes.

The End

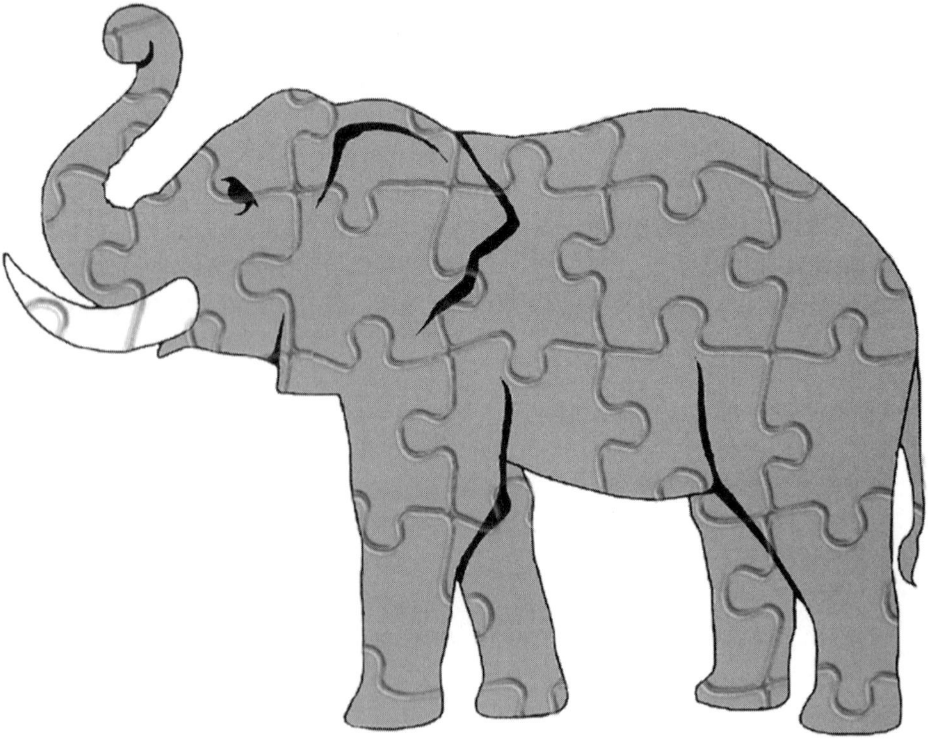

Index

You can be a part of this continuing medical advance

Join IOD with a membership and stay updated
Be at the cutting edge of medical information

Yes, I am happy to help! Here's my tax deductible contribution.

Annual Dues Structure

( ) **Benefactor $10,000-$50,000**
( ) **Patron $5,000-$9,999**
( ) **Sponsor $1,000-$4,999**
( ) **Sustaining $500-$999**
( ) **Membership $50-$499**

NAME ______________________________

ADDRESS ______________________________

CITY ____________________ **ST** ____ **ZIP** __________

PHONE ________________

Visa or MasterCard *(circle one)*

Card # ____________________ *Exp. date* __________

Signature ______________________________

Mail to IOD
433 Westwind Drive
North Palm Beach, FL 33408-5123
561-840-8512

Iod@ironoverload.org
www.ironoverload.org

Fax 561-842-9881

tick...tick...tick...
By Roberta Crawford

"A spellbinding and moving mystery based on mankind's least known disease (iron overload). Intrigue and treachery on a grand scale. A read you won't forget. It may even save your life."
CLIVE CUSSLER
Best-selling Novelist

"The author has put together a racy and fast-moving story at the end of which, almost sub-consciously, the reader will be well educated about the commonest lethal hereditary disease in our population. That is quite an achievement!"
A. BRIAN WEST, MD
Yale University

"This is the first novel I've ever read that could save a person's life."
HAROLD M. BATES, PhD
MetPath Sciences Director